The Spectrum Of Migraine

Case-Based Medicine Teaching Series

McMahon Publishing Group
New York, NY

The McMahon Publishing Group, New York City 2002.

The use of general descriptive names, trade names, trademarks, etc., in this publication, even if the former are not especially identified, is not to be taken as a sign that such names, as understood by the Trade Marks and Merchandise Marks Act, may accordingly be used freely by anyone.

While the advice and information in this book are believed to be true and accurate at the date of going to press, neither the authors nor the editors nor the publisher can accept any legal responsibility for any errors or omissions that may have been made. The publisher makes no warranty, expressed or implied, with respect to material contained herein.

ISBN (0-9641623-4-2)

Typeset by Max Graphics, New York City

Printed in the U.S.A.

The Spectrum of Migraine

Table of Contents

Note From the Editors

While the common denominator is pain and disability, migraine presents in a variety of forms, with a variety of "faces." This variability occurs across and within patients. The same patient can have headaches that sometimes meet diagnostic criteria for migraine without aura, migraine with aura, migrainous headache, episodic tension-type headache, and aura without headache. This has been referred to by Neil Raskin, vice chairman and professor of neurology at University of California, San Francisco, School of Medicine, as "the continuum of benign recurring headache," but we call it the spectrum of migraine.

Migraine can also vary across the population of patients, and can be confused with sinusitis, jaw dysfunction, tension or "stress" headache, neck problems, and other common ailments. Episodic migraine can transform into chronic migraine and daily headache.

This book consists of case descriptions of headache, prepared by headache specialists who range in their training specialty: family practice, internal medicine, dentistry, emergency medicine, and neurology. All of the cases are presented initially without a diagnosis; the diagnosis is then provided during the discussion. Recommended reading selections complete each chapter.

The hope is that physicians will read the case presentations and try to come up with a diagnosis and approach to treatment before reading the discussion. Our goal is to help physicians identify migraine in its many forms, as well as some common headache disorders sharing features with migraine, and to discuss up-to-date management of these headaches.

We hope you enjoy reading these cases and learn from them. The discussions should help you to perfect your own treatment of these headache syndromes.

Stewart J. Tepper, MD
Fred D. Sheftell, MD
Alan M. Rapoport, MD

The New England Center for Headache
Stamford, Connecticut
September 2002

1. The Man With Episodic Disabling Headaches

Alan G. Finkel, MD

Director, University Headache Clinic
University of North Carolina
Chapel Hill, NC

Case

A 44-year-old general internist presented for evaluation of headache dating back to a distinctive memory of a severely disabling headache at 12 years of age.

In college, his headaches would go on for days, with occasional severe and disabling attacks of shorter duration (less than 24 hours).

The patient recalled having headaches on and after call nights during his critical care fellowship (age 28 to 30). By his middle 30s, he was using approximately 20 isometheptene combination medications per month. He awakened with a dull bilateral pain that would "focus" (the patient's words) unilaterally an average of 6 to 9 times per month.

Five years of headache calendars that he brought with him on his initial visit showed an average of 1 to 3 severe unilateral headaches per month. These headaches were precipitated by changes in sleep patterns. He noted that in the hours before a headache, he became "ravenous."

Visual aura never preceded his attacks, and his headaches were usually associated with profound phonophobia. He tended to seek out darkness, especially shunning fluorescent light, although he did not use the word "photophobia."

The patient never ate during the hours of severe pain, but he did not have frank nausea. On rare occasions, he did vomit. He had no history of car sickness, although he did not like roller coasters even as an adult.

The headaches resolved with administration of sumatriptan (Imitrex) 25 mg, but the patient was never headache-free after the first dose. He used a second dose 75% of the time, which always resulted in a pain-free state. Preventive medications tried in the past included propranolol, amitriptyline, fluoxetine, divalproex sodium (Depakote), verapamil, and, most recently, a COX-II inhibitor and magnesium.

Past Medical History

Remarkable for familial tremor and childhood asthma. Alcohol consumption consisted of 1 cocktail per week (although he abstained during headaches).

Family History

Remarkable for paternal migraine, depression, and Parkinson's disease. Members of his family remembered no family history of heart disease or stroke before the age of 50. The subject had one brother with major depressive disorder. His 10-year-old daughter required periodic treatment for headache.

Systems Review

Remarkable for whiplash at the age of 30, with resultant chronic neck pain. The man exercised daily. He described difficulty falling asleep and early-morning awakening. When asked about his mood, he stated, "With my headaches, I guess I'm getting by."

Exam

His general exam was unremarkable, and neurologic exam was nonfocal and nonlateralizing. Tenderness was noted in the temporalis, masseter, and fronto-occipitalis muscles.

Discussion

This man has migraine without aura, the understanding and treatment of which constitute the heart and soul of headache medicine. The characteristics and associated features of the headache in migraine without aura, as recognized by the International Headache Society (IHS) criteria, are identical to those in migraine attacks associated with aura. Anecdotally, patients who suffer both have greater dread of migraines without aura, describing them as more disabling, often with more intense pain. Like migraine with aura, migraine without aura is female predominant, more prevalent through the productive and childbearing years, and inversely proportional to income.

Our first task is to try to understand what occurs in migraine without aura. In aura, there are clearly discernible, reversible neurologic events. However, when a patient suffers a migraine without aura, it is assumed that the cerebrum is sensitive to changes in the internal and external environments superimposed on a genetic (or, less often, acquired) neural substrate. The brain of migraine patients is thus described as hyperexcitable or oversensitive.

Migraine pain occurs after exposure to a variety of triggers. The migraine brain sensitivity predisposes the patient to these triggers by sensitizing the brain and brain stem, initiating the series of events that result in migraine.

The brain firing that initiates migraine pain probably starts in cortical and subcortical areas, possibly in a "midbrain generator." This, in turn, stimulates trigeminovascular structures, activating peripheral pain mechanisms in the meninges such as inflammatory change and vasodilation. This peripheral nociceptive pain mechanism, in turn, sensitizes trigeminal pain afferents, which transduce the pain signal centrally. This results in pain in the head, upper face, and occipitonuchal areas.

The most common triggers are disruptions to those chronobiologic constants of sleep excess or deprivation, hunger, and stress (either in its "buildup" or "letdown" phase). Modulation of the pain experience occurs in other brain-stem areas, while secondary stimulation of cranial and extracranial structures maintains the pain experience. This experience can also be manifested as tension-type or sinus headache (the 2 most common misdiagnoses of migraine without aura).

Central processing of the pain, in turn, activates autonomic nuclei and systems with generation of migraine-associated symptoms, including nausea, photophonophobia, and dysautonomia. With resolution of pain, it should be expected that the associated features and migraine-associated disability also abate. From these basic understandings have come extraordinary advances in the acute and preventive management of migraine without aura.

Establishing Risk for Disease

Migraine without aura occurs in males at a rate of 6%, with a peak prevalence at age 30 to 39 years. For females, a peak incidence year of 15 establishes a population prevalence peaking in the late 30s to mid-40s, with an overall prevalence of 18%. Before the development of headache associated with migraine attacks, preadolescents may have motion sickness, episodic vertigo, vomiting, abdominal pain, or brief, self-limited headache. The singular memory of a headache in this patient (which is common in migraine patients) should be taken as a sign of its severity, since memory of childhood events is usually significant.

Headaches of longer duration that present during the transitional years of education (18 to 28) reflect not only the maturation of the disease but also the influence that disordered lifestyles (eg, sleep pattern abnormalities, recreational activities including alcohol use and strenuous mental and physical activities) impart upon this condition. The inability to elicit a history of aura is probably accurate, since aura is a startling and memorable experience. The declining incidence after 40 to 49 years reflects the many life changes that occur (hormonal, social/familial, general health).

The presence of medical comorbidities is another important component of the migraine complex. Migraine sufferers have greater relative risks for many medical conditions, including asthma, irritable bowel syndrome, familial tremor, epilepsy, and stroke. In addition, it is now well established that migraine without aura shares 2 very important comorbidities with aura-associated migraine: affective disease (depression, anxiety) and tension-type headache. The presence of melancholic symptoms, including sleep disturbance and low mood is suggestive, although a drive toward high-level functioning is often seen as the hallmark of the migraine personality (if such an entity exists).

A family history of migraine is seen in 80% of patients, and there is growing evidence for a genetic basis in many forms of migraine. Monogenetic risk for migraine without aura has not been established. Although genes for migraine with aura and familial hemiplegic migraine have been demonstrated at gene loci including 19p13, 1q21-23, and 1q31 (see Aurora chapter, page 105), candidate genes for migraine without aura have recently been suggested at loci including Xq24-28, Xp22, and 4q24.

The presence of depression in patients with familial migraine may be indirect evidence for a predisposition toward migraine in those with no known first- or second-degree relative with migraine. Because acquired migraine may also occur in individuals without prior risk, a detailed history of trauma, including traumatic life events, should be included.

Making the Diagnosis

In its most common form, this primary headache disorder is immediately recognizable, although the variability of presentation is what imparts to "common migraine" the dubious distinction of gross underdiagnosis. The most recent population-based study showed that more than 50% of patients with migraine without aura remain undiagnosed. Our second task, therefore, is to elicit from the patient a reproducible group of descriptors that allow us to "pattern recognize" that the person sitting in front of us has migraine without aura. The limited number of ways in which humans can describe their subjective experience flaws the description of pain and other neurologic phenomena. Thus, the term "sick headache" typifies this obfuscation of common terminology.

Yet even in this patient, one well versed in medical terminology, it is difficult to squeeze his descriptors into a criteria-based classification such as that put forward by the IHS criteria for migraine without aura (Table). The reasons for this are many, but a closer look at the occurrence rates of the features of migraine offers the best opportunity for understanding.

With the use of epidemiologic data, it becomes obvious that if the interviewer is expecting migraine to present with one-sided throbbing pain associated with vomiting, there will be as many as 50% of patients who escape adequate diagnosis. A more specific and sensitive hallmark is the activity-associated worsening of pain in migraine without aura, a finding that has been illustrated in validated assessment instruments that demonstrate unequivocally the importance of disability as a feature and consequence of migraine without aura.

The clinician who seeks location and pain characteristics would do better to ask, "What do you do when you have a headache?" than to pursue a single specific feature such as gastrointestinal disturbance or unilaterality. Those

Table. International Headache Society Migraine Without Aura and Occurrence of Features*

- At least 5 headaches, lasting 4 to 72 hours, with normal exam or imaging study and:

     Characteristics, requiring 2/4:

     Unilateral (40% bilateral or generalized)

     Throbbing (50% nonpulsating)

     Moderate to severe intensity (1% to 2% mild)

     Pain worsened by exertion (<5% not worsened)

- Associated symptoms, requiring 1/2:

     Nausea (5% to 14% not nauseated) or
       vomiting (38% to 70% without vomiting)

     Photophobia (5% to 18% not present) and
       phonophobia (2% to 39% not present)

*Dr. Finkel's comments in parentheses

who respond that they limit or curtail their work, home, or leisure activities during their recurrent headache not only have an extremely high likelihood of migraine but also have a predictably positive response to specific acute migraine therapies in the form of triptans. It is, therefore, incumbent upon the examining clinician to listen closely to the patient and ask questions directed at the reproducible reduction in normal functional activities that almost all sufferers of migraine without aura experience.

Developing a Treatment Plan

The first and most important part of any disease management strategy is to establish the goals of treatment. In order to set these goals, the examiner should elicit triggers, frequency, severity, "time to peak" (of paramount importance in choice of drug and route of administration), prior response to acute and preventive medications (including side effects), and patient preference. A brief educational session is crucial, and has been shown to increase patient satisfaction, enhance treatability, and reduce migraine impact.

Establishing a vocabulary and providing basic information about the disease, including pathophysiology, will allow the clinician to better describe the potential treatment choices. Although migraine without aura does not have an overt cerebral/cortical manifestation, the initiation of migraine may manifest as a noticeable prodrome, occurring up to several hours before the onset of pain. Common prodromes include behavioral excitability, sedation, yawning, hunger, carbohydrate craving (as in this patient), exhaustion, or gastrointestinal symptoms. Describing these to patients often elicits a knowing response, and thus may be used to design early therapies for acute migraine attacks.

Early use of specific migraine medications (eg, triptans) will be more likely to result in fewer and milder side effects, higher pain-free efficacy, and lower recurrence rates. Using the "time-to-peak" intensity and presence or absence of associated symptoms (eg, nausea and vomiting) will help the clinician determine the best route of administration and frequency of acute treatments.

Most patients who seek medical attention for migraine experience impact on their lives, disability, and time loss from their attacks. The Disabilities in Strategies of Care (DISC) study established that patients with disability from their migraines should be treated with triptans for their attacks from the beginning, rather than being stepped up to triptans after failure of lower-level, nonspecific medications. Thus, early use of triptans, both in the course of the migraine illness and in the sequence of an attack, will result in better outcomes for patients with migraine without aura.

Headache calendars help both the clinician and the patient to view, with a more objective eye, the different ways in which migraine without aura manifests in that individual. Many sufferers are surprised at the great frequency of "other" headaches beside the "killers" that they suffer. These milder migraines, migrainous headaches, and episodic tension-type headaches end up being confounders that often lead migraine without aura to be underestimated and underdiagnosed.

The typical pattern of migraine without aura is, on average, 1 or under per month, lasting 24 hours or less, although in patients seen in a headache practice, 1 to 3 migraines without aura per month is more usual. For the person with more frequent attacks, or for those whose acute strategies are failing, preventive management should be given careful consideration.

Most major classes of preventive medications can now be tied to specific receptors or have a suggested mechanism of action that impedes the flow of neuronal information initiating the migraine attack. Thus, most preventive medications reduce the likelihood of brain-stem migraine generator firing.

For these reasons, the more recent additions to the armory of preventives include a growing number of antiepileptic drugs—the goal of which is to provide cortical desensitization without intolerable neuropsychological effects. These monotherapies may also be used to treat psychiatric comorbidities, as the ß-adrenergic and calcium channel blockers may have more utility in patients with mild to moderate and treatable hypertension or cardiac risk. Finally, tricyclic antidepressants, which are useful in migraine prevention, can be used to treat comorbid depression and sleep disorders. Since some patients cannot safely take specific acute antimigraine therapies such as triptans and ergots, the clinician should take these considerations into account when deciding on preventive and maintenance strategies.

In addition, integrative strategies and nonallopathic medications may offer some benefit, although controlled trials and medical evidence are still in the early stages of development. Nevertheless, many patients prefer these "more natural" substances, anticipating potentially fewer side effects. Acceding to patient preference will increase the likelihood of treatment plan compliance. The efficacy of magnesium 400 to 600 mg per day is still in debate (in spite of 5 double-blind, controlled published trials), although it may offer additional benefits to patients who do not develop treatment-related diarrhea. A small but well-designed trial of riboflavin (vitamin B_2) 400 mg/day has established its utility and safety. Feverfew lacks consistent positive evidence, and its long-term efficacy and safety are not established.

Acupuncture appears to work only for acute attack management. Biofeedback is well established as a therapy, especially in the young and for those who are unable to take or tolerate standard medications, and there is some evidence to support the value of cognitive behavioral therapies in long-term use.

Lastly, lifestyle readjustments offer real benefit for those with frequent and disabling migraine without aura. Regular exercise, attention to sleep hygiene, diet, and relaxation/stress management have all been shown to improve the clinical course of migraine without aura. Dietary intake of specific food classes may be overrated as the main cause of increasing migraine without aura, although recognition of specific food triggers should be addressed in the context of these considerations.

The tendency among migraineurs with frequent attacks to limit or curtail enjoyable activities for fear of headache should also be addressed. Telling the patient to increase recreational activities and to have more "fun" offers the clinician an opportunity to discuss the social isolation that many migraine sufferers endure.

Determining Prognosis

All patients deserve a credible diagnosis and prognosis. Complicating prognostication for patients is that migraine actually consists of 2 features: 1) a medical disorder or disease state consisting of a particular brain condition that can result in the triggering or spontaneous onset of recurrent headaches and 2) a headache with associated features. Therefore, in order to discuss prognosis, we should address factors that influence the natural history or life course of the disorder in addition to offering the patient information about the expected results of acute treatment strategies. Management of migraine is disease management; migraine is a chronic, often lifelong illness, making its management not unlike that of hypertension or asthma.

Strict criteria-based diagnosis, although not necessary for the practitioner, has been used in all the clinical trials of triptans throughout the world, and response rates are predictable. In one early study with sumatriptan injection, patients meeting all criteria had a response rate greater than 90%. The typical oral triptan response rates range from approximately 60% to 80%.

Patients with the spectrum of headaches (eg, migraine, migrainous, and tension-type headaches) were shown to respond prospectively to sumatriptan when compared to placebo. Clinically, however, more severe headaches and headaches established over days may have a less complete response to medication. As noted above, there are now strong suggestions that treating each headache as early as possible increases the likelihood that the patient will become pain-free, thus reducing the central sensitization of cranial and extracranial pain-producing structures. The end result of more adequate treatment of acute attacks may, therefore, be one way to reduce the tendency in some patients to become increasingly refractory to treatment, ultimately allowing for progression of the disorder to more frequent, difficult-to-treat headaches.

Offering a long-term prognosis involves other factors and, as in our patient, demands that our attention be diverted to other important components of this neurologic disorder. Genetics and environmental influences may coexist and reduce the likelihood of a positive long-term prognosis. Also, as frequency increases, disabling features may be more prominent, as may neuropsychological complications such as depression and anxiety. Therefore, the patient who proceeds to more frequent headaches may require additional evaluations, including psychological consultation, in addition to a heightened attention to the positive and negative potentials of polytherapy.

Conclusion

Treating migraine without aura offers a great opportunity to benefit patients' quality of life and feeling of well-being. When the illness is associated with significant medical, surgical, or psychological comorbidity, the intellectual challenges for treatment are greater. Still, helping to effect a better outcome and prognosis is tremendously satisfying for the physician. The interested clinician can easily learn better treatment paradigms. Understanding pathophysiology, the current status of migraine epidemiology, and the confounding factors to diagnosing migraine without aura can improve diagnosis and reduce overprescription of inappropriate, nonspecific, habituating medications in multiple classes, including those that engender rebound and daily headaches, or—just as bad—compel progression of disease.

The basic principles, therefore, are:

1. Recurrent, severe headaches that are unassociated with systemic dis-

ease or neurologic complications can be diagnosed as migraine even in the absence of the classically discussed features of aura (unilaterality, associated gastrointestinal symptoms, or throbbing pain).

2. Response to medication may be predicted on the basis of medical evidence, although individual variability and comorbidities should determine safety and preference.
3. Education of the patient will improve compliance and reliability of follow-up information.
4. Objective measures, especially the use of headache calendars, can help determine the need for additional treatments or change in treatment strategy.
5. Prognosis can be determined in patients with migraine without aura. Disease complexity makes this determination more challenging and interesting, requiring attention to genetics, environmental factors, and comorbidities.
6. Progression of disease can be prevented with appropriate migraine-specific (triptan) treatment of acute attacks.
7. Adequate elimination of acute attacks (sustained pain-free response to triptans), avoidance of inadequate, nonspecific acute care medications, and, when appropriate, reduction of attack frequency with appropriate prevention may be the best hope for preventing or reversing migraine progression in the treatable patient.

The treating physician should make every attempt to match his or her treatment goals with the expectations of patients. Issues of health maintenance and recognition of comorbidities become powerful tools for both parties to use in improving outcomes and reducing the tendency toward disease progression.

Editors' Note

Epidemiologic data suggest that 94% of patients complaining of headache to primary care physicians have migraine or migrainous headache. An established pattern (>6 months) of episodic, disabling headache with a normal exam is considered migraine until proven otherwise. Since the impact, disability, or lost time of patients drives the diagnosis, and since triptans optimize outcomes for disabled migraine patients, triptans should be the first line of treatment for migraine patients in the primary care physician's office. Triptans should never be a last-resort treatment or a second or third step in the treatment of a migraine attack. Comorbidity and high frequency of attacks should lead to consideration of preventive therapies. Avoidance of analgesic and other nonspecific acute-care treatments will prevent headache rebound and, as eloquently summarized by Dr. Finkel, progression.

It bears mentioning that the headache history should include questions about the impact of headache on the patient's life. Dr. Finkel's patient stated, "… I guess I'm getting by." Such instruments as the Migraine Disability Assessment Scale and the Headache Impact Test are useful in quantifying impact.

<u>Diagnosis:</u> **Migraine Without Aura**

Selected Reading

Breslau N, Rasmussen BK. The impact of migraine: epidemiology, risk factors and co-morbidities. *Neurology.* 2001;56:S4-S12.

Lipton RB, Stewart WF, Stone AM, Lainez MJA, Sawyer JPC. The disabilities in strategies of care study: stratified care vs step care strategies for migraine. *JAMA.* 2000;284:2599-2605.

Lipton RB, Stewart WF, Diamond S, Diamond ML, Reed M. Prevalence and burden of migraine in the United States: data from the American Migraine Study II. *Headache.* 2001;41:646-657.

Merikangas KR, Dartigues JF, Whitaker A, Angst J. Diagnostic criteria for migraine: a validity study. *Neurology.* 1994:44:S11-S16.

Osterhaus JT, Townsend RJ, Gandek B, Ware JE. Measuring the functional status and well-being of patients with migraine headache. *Headache.* 1994;34:337-343.

Solomon GD. Evolution of the measurement of quality of life in migraine. *Neurology.* 1997:48:S10-S15.

US Headache Consortium. Multispecialty Consensus on Diagnosis and Treatment of Headache: "Headache Guidelines." *www.aan.com.*

2. The Woman With Low-Level Headaches

Robert Kaniecki, MD

Director, The Headache Center
Assistant Professor of Neurology
University of Pittsburgh
Pittsburgh, Pennsylvania

Case

Ellen is a 40-year-old flight attendant who consulted for a 20-year history of recurrent headaches.

The patient reported the initial development of headaches during college; she particularly recalled more frequent episodes near the time of midterm or final examinations. After graduation, she worked briefly in retail sales until she became a flight attendant for a major commercial airline. During the past 10 years as a senior flight attendant, she has noted a number of triggers for these headaches aside from stress, including sleep deprivation, skipped meals, and, occasionally, barometric pressure changes. Transatlantic flights (bringing changes in her sleep and meal patterns) and even routes from the New York City area to Florida (producing high stress levels) have been particularly problematic with regard to headache frequency.

Ellen described a variable frequency of headache, ranging from 1 to 4 episodes per month. Over the past 2 years, since the birth of her second child and the introduction of additional stressors in her work environment, she has experienced an escalation in frequency to 2 to 3 episodes per week.

Despite the increased frequency, the headache characteristics, duration, and response to therapy have not changed significantly. Each attack tends to begin with a sense of "tightness" bilaterally in the occipital area; within 1 to 2 hours, she has a "heavy cap" of pressure surrounding her cranium.

The discomfort is described as steady, moderate in intensity, and generally relieved by significant distraction or physical activity. Ellen finds herself occasionally sensitive to loud noise, but denies any sensitivity to light, odor, or motion. There is neither nausea nor vomiting, and aside from the cervical discomfort, there is no clear evidence of prodrome, aura, or postdrome. Untreated attacks last approximately 8 to 12 hours.

Generally, Ellen experiences relief after strenuous physical activity, analgesic intake, or sleep. If the headache continues to build throughout the day, it may actually settle in a hemicranial distribution and develop a mild, throbbing character. Simple analgesics taken at this stage tend to be only partly effective, and instead of working within 1 hour, they may take 2 to 3 hours to have an effect. Because of the progression in frequency over the past 12 to 24 months, Ellen now presents for evaluation of these headaches.

Past Medical History, Allergies, and Habits

Otherwise notable only for mild exertional asthma and 2 vaginal vertex deliveries. She has an allergy to penicillin and currently is taking a prescription monophasic oral contraceptive. There was no significant alcohol or tobacco history, but she did mention modest intake of caffeine (2 or 3 8-ounce cups of coffee per day).

Medications

Ellen usually treated the headaches with a nonprescription form of naproxen sodium, dosed at 440 mg once or twice daily, as needed.

Family and Social History

Positive for a mother with headache (similar in quality and reduced after menopause).

Review of Systems

Notable for mild difficulties falling asleep and a sense of mild, generalized anxiety. Ellen specifically denied motion sensitivity, "ice cream" headaches (sensitivity to cold), depression, panic attacks, prior head trauma, or symptoms of irritable bowel syndrome.

General Medical Examination

Completely normal. The subject's pulse was 74, and her blood pressure was 126/72. Her cardiac exam revealed a regular rate and rhythm and normal sounds without the presence of any midsystolic click. There was mild tightness and tenderness in the paraspinal cervical musculature bilaterally, and a slight click at the left temporomandibular joint without pain. Full range was noted at both the cervical and temporomandibular joint levels.

Neurologic Examination

Completely normal, aside from evidence of a minimal bilateral upper extremity postural tremor.

Discussion

Ellen presents with a history and examination consistent with the diagnosis of episodic tension-type headache (ETTH). She describes a 20-year history of episodes of moderate-intensity headache pain lasting 12 hours.

These headaches meet complete International Headache Society (IHS) diagnostic criteria (Table 1, page 23) for ETTH. Aside from being moderate in intensity, the pain is usually bilateral, steady, and without aggravation by routine physical activity. Ellen experiences neither nausea nor vomiting, and has only phonophobia as an associated symptom. While she does describe occasional prolonged attacks as unilateral or mildly pulsatile, these features do not preclude the diagnosis.

Her history has shown some progression in headache frequency over 2 years, and although her headache features are quite stable, this fundamental change in headache pattern should serve as a "red flag" to consider the presence of an organic etiology. Her examination is notable for some cervical muscular tightness and tenderness, which may be seen in patients with tension-type headache. The additional presence of a mild postural tremor should provoke consideration of anxiety or organic conditions such as caffein-ism and hyperthyroidism. In this case, a magnetic resonance image of the brain with and without gadolinium, in conjunction with routine serum studies includ-ing thyroid function tests, would be appropriate.

Ellen presents with a relatively characteristic description of ETTH. At this point, the clinical characteristics, epidemiology, pathophysiology, and man-agement of ETTH will be discussed, and specific attention will be paid to the clinical overlap with migraine headaches.

Clinical Characteristics of ETTH

ETTH is the most frequent, but least distinct, of all the primary headache disorders. A diagnosis of tension-type headache by IHS criteria is based chiefly on negative characteristics. Whereas migraine is characterized pri-marily by the presence of "positive" features of photophobia or phonopho-bia, nausea and vomiting, and pain worsening with activity, the IHS classification characterizes tension-type headache by the absence of these features (Table 1).

Tension-type headaches are divided into episodic and chronic subtypes, with the episodic subtype involving attacks on fewer than 15 days per month or 180 days per year. By definition, these headaches may last from 30 min-utes to 7 days.

As opposed to the unilateral, throbbing, moderate to severe pain of migraine, tension-type headache is characterized by bilateral, steady, and mild to moderate pain qualities. There is no prodrome, aura, or postdrome. The episodes usually begin during daytime hours, and patients frequently describe escalation throughout the day. The headache is generally associated with min-imal disability. Physical activity generally has minimal impact on headache intensity. Occasionally patients will report slight photophobia or phonophobia, scalp tenderness, or muscular tension or soreness in the cervical region. The most common precipitating factors mentioned include stress and sleep dis-ruption. Aside from the use of analgesic therapy, common palliative measures include rest or sleep, physical massage or manipulation, local application of heat or ice, and sometimes aerobic exercise.

The IHS subclassifies ETTH into categories with and without disorder of per-icranial musculature, which may include increased muscle contraction or ten-derness. Certain patients may have points or bands of muscular tension and soreness that may be detected by manual palpation of both the pericranial and cervical areas. Both between and during headache attacks, patients with ten-sion-type headache have more muscle tenderness than do nonheadache con-trols. Abnormal electromyographic activity may be identified in some patients.

Because of the paucity of associated features and the lack of severe pain or disability, ETTH rarely is a presenting complaint. It is imperative to exclude the possibility of a secondary headache disorder in a child or adult who pre-sents with headaches suggestive of a tension-type picture. Headaches with similar characteristics are commonly seen in patients presenting with eleva-tions in intracranial pressure, such as that seen with brain tumor, pseudo-tumor cerebri, or hydrocephalus. Although the nondescript nature of tension-type headaches may suggest a relatively benign presentation, one must be vigilant for specific "red flags" for organic disease.

Since, by definition, ETTH is neither severe nor frequent, a crucial question to ask any patient with this presentation is "What provoked you to come to the office?" Particularly worrisome features are new presentations of such headaches in individuals younger than age 5 or older than age 50, past history of cancer or immunosuppression, exacerbation with physical activity or Valsalva's maneuver, or fundamental change in headache pattern. In such instances, neuroimaging studies and other investigations should be added to a detailed neurologic examination.

Epidemiology

Tension-type headache is the most common primary or secondary headache, with prevalence ranging from 30% to 80% in population-based studies. In a Danish study (Iversen et al), the lifetime prevalence for tension-type headache was 69% in men and 88% in women, with a 1-year prevalence of 63% in men and 86% in women. More recent estimates place the prevalence of IHS-defined ETTH at 40% in the adult population. There is a slight female preponderance, with a female-to-male ratio of 1.2:1 to 1.6:1 in studies performed in Denmark and the United States, respectively. Prevalence of tension-type headache peaks between the ages of 30 and 39, and subsequently declines with age in both sexes. There is also a correlation between increased prevalence of tension-type headache and higher educational levels.

Pathophysiology

The origin of tension-type headache was initially proposed as arising from excessive contraction of pericranial and cervical muscles, leading to one of the original terms of "muscle contraction headache." Many believe a link exists between these headaches and emotional distress or "life tension." Studies have been unable to establish any clear correlation among muscle contraction, soreness, or tenderness and the presence of headache.

It has been postulated that tension-type headache arises from abnormal neuronal sensitivity and facilitation of pain transmission. The trigeminal nucleus caudalis in the brain stem acts as the major sensory relay center for all pain signals of the head and upper neck, where input from intracranial and extracranial structures converges. Neurons in this nucleus may be sensitized secondary to excessive activation of myofascial nociceptors, while primary disorders of central pain modulation may also be present.

Overlap With Migraine

The difficulty in distinguishing ETTH from migraine headache, 2 of the most common episodic headache types, is widely acknowledged. Among respondents in the American Migraine Study II who met IHS criteria for migraine but who lacked a physician diagnosis of migraine, 32% reported a physician diagnosis of tension-type headache.

Moreover, in a recently reported post hoc analysis of data from the Spectrum Study, 37% of patients initially diagnosed with tension-type headache were later revealed, on the basis of a neurologist's evaluation of headache diaries and medical records, to have migraine or migrainous headache. Physicians are likely to diagnose tension-type headache when bilateral or non-throbbing head pain is present, if the patient reports that the headache is triggered by stress or muscle tension, or when neck pain is present. In fact, migraine is often associated with these features. In recent studies, 41% of migraineurs reported bilateral pain; more than 50% reported nonpulsating pain; and 84% identified stress or tension as a precipitant of headache.

Neck pain is also quite common in migraine patients. In a recent study of 144 patients meeting IHS criteria for migraine, 75% described neck pain associated with their migraine attacks. Although these patients met IHS criteria for migraine, 82% of them had a previous diagnosis of tension-type headache. Triptans, agonists at the 5-HT$_{1B/1D}$ receptors, have been found to be effective for the tension headache–like symptom of neck pain when it occurred as a feature of migraine in IHS-diagnosed migraineurs.

The similarities between migraine and tension-type headache have led many to question the distinctions between them. The question of whether migraine and tension-type headache are separate disorders or manifestations of the same disorder has been debated for years. Proponents of the continuum-severity theory contend that tension-type headache and migraine constitute the same entity, distinguished only by severity. Proponents of an alternative hypothesis known as the "convergence theory" (see Cady chapter, page 27) contend that tension-type headache and migraine may constitute the same entity, but are distinguished by duration or extent of activation of the central nervous system pain transmission pathways. Others continue to support the concept that tension-type headache and migraine are distinct entities with different pathophysiology and are effectively treated by different therapies. Nevertheless, clinicians providing care for patients with headache should be aware of diagnostic and therapeutic overlaps between these 2 disorders and be cognizant of the implications for the management of patients with headache.

Treatment and Management

The approach to the management of ETTH involves a combination of lifestyle and physical and pharmacologic measures. Recommendations for regulation of sleep, meals, and exercise are generally quite valuable.

Stress management techniques and other steps toward trigger avoidance may be of great benefit. Passive physical manipulation and active cervical muscle stretching or exercise programs are often advised. Behavioral therapies are quite useful adjuncts in the management of ETTH, with the most frequently suggested techniques involving relaxation therapy and electromyogram-guided biofeedback. Cognitive behavioral therapy may provide additional benefit in cases of significant depression or anxiety.

Preventive pharmacologic therapy is generally advised for patients experiencing at least 2 to 3 headache days each week (Table 2, page 24). Although analgesics may continue to be beneficial when taken at such levels, the issues of analgesic rebound and transformation into more refractory cases of chronic tension-type headache must be considered. Progression in frequency or severity of attacks, development of adverse events with acute medications, and decline in efficacy of acute medications may all be additional indications for the institution of daily pharmacologic preventive therapy.

Although there is little well-controlled scientific evidence to support their use in these headaches, most clinicians advise using antidepressants and anticonvulsants to help stabilize tension-type headaches. Centrally acting muscle relaxants, benzodiazepines, and, lately, botulinum toxin A (Botox) injection have been helpful in individual cases. There is no evidence that standard muscle relaxant therapies are effective in the treatment of these headaches.

Acute therapies are warranted in the majority of tension-type headache cases (Table 3, page 25). They are provided to relieve the pain of individual headache attacks. Simple analgesics, nonsteroidal anti-inflammatory drugs, the newer COX-2 inhibitor nonsteroidal analgesics, and combination agents are most commonly used. Their use should be strictly limited to an average of 2 to 3 days per week at most, to avoid the issues of analgesic rebound and potential contribution toward transformation into chronic tension-type headache. Opioid analgesics are rarely, if ever, necessary to control this type of headache.

Should the investigation yield no significant findings, a treatment program for this patient should be designed to directly address tension-type headaches. Nonpharmacologic steps would involve attempts at regulating her sleep, meals, and exercise, particularly noting precipitating factors of

Table 1. Criteria for Episodic Tension-Type Headache

A. At least 10 previous headache episodes fulfilling criteria B-D listed below
   Number of days with such headache <180/year (<15/month)

B. Headache lasting from 30 minutes to 7 days

C. At least 2 of the following pain characteristics:
   • Pressing/tightening (nonpulsating) quality
   • Mild or moderate intensity (may inhibit, but does not prohibit, activity)
   • Bilateral location
   • No aggravation through climbing stairs or similar routine physical activity

D. Both of the following:
   • No nausea or vomiting (anorexia may still occur)
   • Photophobia and phonophobia are absent, or one but not the other is present

E. History, physical, or neurologic examination normal

sleep and meal deprivation. Caffeine and stress reduction should be addressed, and biofeedback or relaxation training should be instituted.

Given the escalation in headache frequency to a level of 2 to 3 attacks per week, daily preventive therapy should be strongly considered. Considering the presence of comorbid mild anxiety and insomnia, low doses of antidepressants (tricyclics, selective serotonin reuptake inhibitors) might prove beneficial.

Since naproxen sodium tends to be largely effective for this patient at a dose of 440 mg once or twice daily, the dose should be increased to the prescription strength of 550 mg to provide coverage for more intense episodes. Regardless of whether daily preventive therapy is initiated, the use of analgesic therapy must be strictly monitored by a headache diary to prevent the development of overuse and associated "rebound" headaches.

Editors' Note

Tension-type headache is a "featureless" headache, and is characterized by being "not migraine." In proposed new criteria for the IHS, all features of migraine are eliminated from the definition of tension-type headache: it is not unilateral, not throbbing, not made worse with routine physical activity, not severe, and not associated with nausea, photophobia, or phonophobia.

Table 2. Preventive Treatments for Frequent Episodic Tension-Type Headaches

Tricyclic antidepressants

Amitriptyline (Elavil)	10-250 mg/d
Desipramine (Norpramin)	10-200 mg/d
Doxepin (Sinequan)	10-200 mg/d
Nortriptyline (Aventyl)	10-150 mg/d

Selective serotonin reuptake inhibitors

Fluoxetine (Prozac)	10-40 mg/d
Paroxetine (Paxil)	10-40 mg/d
Sertraline (Zoloft)	25-200 mg/d

Other agents

Baclofen (Lioresal)	10-80 mg/d
Clonazepam (Klonopin)	0.5-3 mg/d
Divalproex sodium (Depakote)	500-2,000 mg/d
Gabapentin (Neurontin)	600-2,400 mg/d
Nefazodone (Serzone)	50-600 mg/d
Tizanidine (Zanaflex)	2-20 mg/d
Venlafaxine (Effexor)	37.5-300 mg/d

This featureless presentation makes both the pathophysiology obscure and the treatment necessarily empiric. Dr. Kaniecki provides a convenient, commonsense approach for the management of this usually mild nuisance headache.

Most patients do not complain to the primary physician about tension-type headache unless it is very frequent. Most ETTH is not disabling. The presence of an established pattern of episodic disabling headache with normal exam should be considered migraine, not ETTH, until proven otherwise.

However, as Dr. Kaniecki points out and as is discussed in the Cady (page 27) and Tepper (page 38) chapters, migraine patients often present with a spectrum of headache with phenotypic ETTH at one end, and these tension-type headaches in migraine patients are probably just low-level migraines, responsive to sumatriptan (Imitrex) or other triptans, and represent one end of a continuum. It is the editors' opinion that tension-type headache is likely a heterogeneous disorder, which may be on the continuum with migraine and sometimes related to myofascial mechanisms.

In Table 3, Dr. Kaniecki lists many reasonable analgesics that can be tried for occasional relief of episodic tension-type headache. However, we would like to emphasize his earlier point on a preference for prudent, low-frequen-

Table 3. Acute Treatments for Episodic Tension-Type Headaches

Simple Analgesics

Acetaminophen	650-1,000 mg qid
Acetylsalicylic acid (ASA)	650-1,000 mg qid
Celecoxib (Celebrex)	100-200 mg bid
Ibuprofen	400-800 mg tid
Ketoprofen	50-75 mg qid
Naproxen	220-550 mg bid
Rofecoxib (Vioxx)	12.5-50 mg qd
Valdecoxib (Bextra)	10-40 mg qd

Combination Analgesics

ASA/acetaminophen/caffeine	2 tabs qid
Butalbital compounds	1-2 tabs qid
Isometheptene compounds	1 tab qid (or 2 + 2)

Other Agents

Clonazepam (Klonopin)	0.25-1 mg bid
Codeine	15-60 mg qid
Tramadol (Ultram)	50-100 mg qid

cy use: Even though Table 3 lists up to 1 tablet of a given medication qid, the patient must limit intake of acute care medications to 2 or 3 days a week, and list usage in a headache diary. Otherwise, as Dr. Kaniecki points out, there is a likelihood of inducing analgesic rebound headache or medical problems related to overuse syndromes.

<u>Diagnosis:</u> Episodic Tension-Type Headache

Selected Reading

Dahlof CGH, Jacobs LD. Ketoprofen, paracetamol and placebo in the treatment of episodic tension-type headache. *Cephalalgia.* 1996;16:117-123.

Davidoff RA. Trigger points and myofascial pain: toward understanding how they affect headaches. *Cephalalgia.* 1998;18:436-448.

Hatch JP, Moore PJ, Cyr-Provost M, et al. The use of electromyography and muscle palpation in the diagnosis of tension-type headache with and without pericranial muscle involvement. *Pain.* 1992;49:175-178.

Headache Classification Committee of the International Headache Society. Classification and diagnostic criteria for headache disorders, cranial neuralgias and facial pain. *Cephalalgia.* 1988;8(suppl 7):196.

Iversen HK, Langemark M, Andersson PG, Hansen PE, Olesen J. Clinical characteristics of migraine and episodic tension-type headache in relation to old and new diagnostic criteria. *Headache.* 1990;30:514-519.

Jensen R, Bendtsen L, Olesen J. Muscular factors are of importance in tension-type headache. *Headache.* 1998;38:10-17.

Kaniecki RG. Migraine and tension-type headache: an assessment of challenges in diagnosis. *Neurology.* 2002;58(suppl 6):S15-S20.

Lipton RB, Stewart WF, Cady R, et al. Sumatriptan for the range of headaches in migraine sufferers: results of the spectrum study. *Headache.* 2000;40:783-791.

Olesen J. Clinical and pathophysiological observations in migraine and tension-type headache explained by integration of vascular, supraspinal and myofascial inputs. *Pain.* 1991;46:125-132.

Rasmussen BK. Migraine and tension-type headache in a general population: precipitating factors, female hormones, sleep patterns and relation to lifestyle. *Pain.* 1993;53:65-72.

Rasmussen BK, Jensen R, Schroll M, Olesen J. Epidemiology of headache in a general population—a prevalence study. *J Clin Epidemiol.* 1991;44:1147-1157.

Schwartz BS, Stewart WF, Simon D, et al. Epidemiology of tension-type headache. *JAMA.* 1998;279:381-383.

3. The Man With Long-Lasting, Severe Headaches

Roger K. Cady, MD

Director,
Headache Care Center
Founder/Director,
Primary Care Network
Springfield, Mo.

Case

A 37-year-old man presented with the complaint of recurrent headaches.

The headaches had begun in his early 20s as infrequent episodes that often occurred after he "had been out with friends." These occasional headaches were controlled with aspirin or ibuprofen and rest.

His reason for seeking evaluation was that 10 months previously, he had received a promotion at work that necessitated national and international travel. The headaches became more frequent and, because of the demands of his new position, more of a disruption. Even though the subject had not missed work, he often struggled through the day and found it difficult to concentrate during meetings.

The headaches began at the back of his neck and in the suboccipital area. They slowly intensified over several hours until the pain became moderate or even severe. The pain eventually extended into both temples and occasionally behind both eyes, had a steady deep pressure and nonpulsating quality, and was not necessarily aggravated by activity. The subject reported anorexia but no nausea. When the pain was severe, he was sensitive to light and—to a lesser degree—sound. At times the headaches were severe enough for him to want to lie down, but he "forced" himself to finish work before seeking rest. Between episodes of headache, he felt well.

Before 8 months ago, his headaches had occurred 5 or 6 times per year, but over the last 8 months they had increased to 3 or 4 times a month. The headaches lasted 24 to 36 hours and often resolved after deep sleep. The subject expressed fear that the headaches would continue to become more frequent, resulting in further interference with his work.

He typically initiated treatment with various over-the-counter (OTC) medications. If the headache progressed and moved into the temples, he would increase the doses of OTC agents beyond those recommended on the label. He repeated doses of medication every 3 to 4 hours until the headache resolved or he fell asleep. The man felt the medications "took the edge off" his headaches and allowed him to function. Recently, he had been using an OTC product with caffeine, as he felt it helped him stay more alert and think better.

After the headaches resolved, he felt tired, and the muscles in his neck were sore and stiff. Factors that seemed to be associated with the headaches were stress, travel, lack of sleep, and, perhaps, alcohol.

Medical History

The subject reported that he was in excellent health. He had no history of head trauma.

Medications

He was on no other medications except the OTC medications for headache and a daily multivitamin.

Habits

The subject tried to exercise regularly, did not smoke, and drank infrequently and in moderation.

Family History

The subject was adopted.

Previous Workup

The subject had been evaluated for headaches 4 months earlier by a neurologist, and underwent many tests, including magnetic resonance imaging; all results were reported as normal, and he was given a diagnosis of "severe tension headache." The man was reportedly advised that he needed to decrease his workload and exercise more. He was prescribed cyclobenzaprine and a codeine-containing analgesic to use if the OTC medication was ineffective. However, he discontinued both prescriptions because of sedation and interference with cognition.

Exam

His physical and neurologic examinations, conducted when the patient did not have a headache, yielded normal results. His Migraine Disability Assessment Score was 42 (severe impairment), and his Headache Impact Test (HIT)-6 score was 62 (also severe impairment). His Zung Self-Rating Depression Scale score was 18.

Diagnosis and Management Plan

This patient was diagnosed as having migrainous headaches. In all likelihood he had migraine, but his use of OTC medications probably prevented all headache-associated symptoms from evolving. Migrainous headache was described to the patient as a biologic disorder.

Risk factors of travel and sleep cycle disruption were discussed, and travel behaviors that disrupted his circadian clock, including alcohol consumption during airline flights, were emphasized. The patient was prescribed 50 mg of sumatriptan (Imitrex), and was instructed to take the medication early in the headache process, when the headache was still mild. Use of OTC medications was discontinued, as they had already been proven ineffective.

Goals of therapy were established that emphasized preservation of function. These included being pain-free and functioning normally within 2 hours of treatment. The patient was given rescue options of repeating sumatriptan administration at 2 hours if the therapeutic goal was not achieved. He was further advised that should treatment not effectively abort his headache, he should initiate sumatriptan 100 mg at the onset of subsequent migrainous headaches. Finally, he was prescribed and instructed on the use of sumatriptan injection for rescue, abrupt-onset headaches, or, if circumstances demanded, rapid resolution of his headache. He agreed to keep an electronic calendar of his headache pattern on his Palm Pilot and record therapeutic outcomes.

During a 6-week follow-up evaluation, it was revealed that the subject had successfully treated 4 headache episodes with a single dose of sumatriptan 50 mg. He was using an early intervention strategy and had achieved a 2-hour pain-free outcome in 3 of the 4 headache episodes. For the headache in which he had not successfully achieved this goal, the subject reported that treatment was delayed, and recognized that this meant a slower return to normal functioning. He expressed confidence in his treatment program and felt he was adjusting better to his work schedule. Although the subject had not used the injectable form of sumatriptan, he expressed interest in having it available.

During this visit, the patient was advised that if he began to consistently require acute treatment medications for headache more than 2 days a week or if he did not achieve his treatment goals, he should make an appointment to be re-evaluated for prophylactic daily medications. He scheduled a routine follow-up at 6 months.

Discussion

This patient presented with a moderate to severe episodic headache that was nonthrobbing, bilateral, and not aggravated by routine activity. It did, however, limit function. The patient experienced no nausea or vomiting, but developed photophobia and phonophobia. The episodes lasted 24 to 36 hours; similar headaches have recurred in this patient more than 5 times in the past. There was no history of aura or evidence of underlying disease.

Diagnostically, the patient did not fulfill the International Headache Society (IHS) criteria for migraine with or without aura, or tension-type headache. The headache was a primary headache, was clinically significant and disabling, and warranted medical evaluation and therapy.

From a formal diagnostic standpoint, this headache appeared to manifest symptoms that placed it somewhere between migraine and tension-type headache. The pain was generally moderate but at times became severe. The headache did not pulsate, nor was it aggravated by routine activities. It was also bilateral. The lack of unilaterality, aggravation with activity, and pulsatile quality precluded a formal diagnosis of migraine.

On the other hand, it was associated with both photophobia and phonophobia, which precluded the diagnosis of episodic tension-type headache. The diagnostic evaluation was complicated by the fact that this subject was treating his headaches with OTC medications that were likely masking the true symptom evolution of the headache.

One could approach this case more scientifically by offering the patient a diary and asking him to delay treatment for several hours so that a better evaluation of symptoms could be ascertained. However, it is unlikely he would comply, and since the treatment of migrainous headache is the same as for migraine, this evidence-based approach is unnecessary—at least from a pragmatic and humanistic viewpoint.

Fine-Tuning the Diagnosis

From the perspective of the IHS, the diagnosis in this case is migrainous headache. The criteria for migrainous headache are the same as those for migraine without aura *minus 1* diagnostic symptom. Had the headache in this case had any additional IHS-determined qualities (unilateral, aggravated with activity, pulsatile quality), it would have achieved the symptomatology necessary for a migraine diagnosis. On the other hand, if it had demonstrated 1 less symptom (for example, no photophobia), it could have been diagnosed as a tension-type headache. Given the often divergent treatments utilized for acute episodes of migraine versus tension-type headache, exploring the impact of the headache and the probable role of the subject's treatment efforts is valuable.

Category 1 of the IHS classification is migraine. The IHS migrainous headache diagnosis is coded as 1.7 and, as such, is considered a migraine-type headache. From a clinical perspective, this permits clinicians to diagnose headache attacks that have most of the features of migraine but not enough symptoms for a formal IHS diagnosis of migraine. The IHS does not specifically define characteristics of migrainous headache; consequently, physicians have some latitude in defining migrainous headache as distinguished from migraine without aura (IHS 1.1). It should be kept in mind that according to the IHS, any headache following an aura is migraine regardless of headache characteristics or associated symptoms.

The incidence of migrainous headache in the United States has increased significantly over the past decade. Migrainous headache may be experienced as the dominant migraine presentation in a patient. More frequently, migrainous headache is one of many migraine presentations in individuals who experience IHS migraine without aura. In either scenario, patients experiencing these headaches are frequently misdiagnosed and, more important, inadequately treated.

Individuals experiencing migrainous headache may be misdiagnosed because of the symptomatology they experience. In a recent study of subjects with self-described "sinus headaches," 97% met criteria for migraine diagnosis at clinical interview. However, one third of those obtaining a migraine diagnosis fulfilled criteria for migrainous headache rather than migraine without aura. In a second, even larger follow-up study of physician-diagnosed "sinus headache," a similar result was noted. In these populations with migraine and migrainous headache carrying a diagnosis of "sinus headache," a high degree of autonomic symptomatology was observed (nasal congestion and rhinorrhea). While these symptoms are clearly described as being observed in migraine, they are not a formal part of the IHS diagnostic criteria.

Kaniecki recently reported similar results in a population of diagnosed migraine patients who experienced neck and muscle pain as a component of their migraine episodes. In his study, three quarters of those who met criteria for migraine according to a detailed clinical history had previously received a tension headache diagnosis.

Finally, in the recently completed Landmark Study, primary care physicians' diagnoses were compared to those of a panel of headache experts. It was noted that with a diagnosis of migraine, there was a 98% agreement between primary care physicians and headache specialists. However, when primary care physicians made a nonmigraine diagnosis, 82% of these patients were diagnosed by headache experts as having migraine. This underscores the specificity of the IHS migraine definition, but again suggests that sensitivity is lacking because of the narrow symptom inclusion in the diagnostic scheme. To that point, many symptoms commonly noted during migraine, such as neck muscle pain or autonomic symptoms, appear to obscure migraine diagnosis.

Understanding the Complexities of IHS Migraine Diagnosis

The accepted diagnostic criteria for primary headache disorders were established by the IHS in 1988. These criteria were drafted through consensus of a committee of recognized headache experts. As such, these criteria are not evidence-based. The IHS criteria are used to diagnose each episode of headache independently, defining attacks of headache rather than patients with headaches. These criteria were created in anticipation of worldwide clinical trials of medications and were designed to have a high specificity for the acute attack of migraine. This was an important attribute of the IHS criteria for getting triptans approved by multiple regulatory agencies.

However, IHS criteria for migraine have a low sensitivity for migraine. In fact, by the time enough symptoms have emerged for the diagnosis of migraine to be formally made, the pathologic process of migraine is sufficiently advanced that most individuals are significantly impaired. This lack of clinical sensitivity is undoubtedly a factor in the slow adoption of the IHS diagnostic criteria into clinical practice.

Further, adherence to IHS diagnostic criteria requires multiple primary headache diagnoses for many, if not most, patients. In turn, if there are different diagnoses, it is easy to assume there should be different treatments. Adding to the confusion is the fact that in clinical practice, headache histories obtained from patients may be distorted through self-treatment efforts, obscuring symptoms that would be present had treatment been sufficiently delayed. For example, use of an OTC product may keep headache from throbbing or being aggravated by activity. These factors are important contributors to the misdiagnosis and mismanagement of migraine.

Defining the Boundaries of Primary Headache

Migraine is a complex neurobiologic disorder. Headache is generally a prominent symptom that emerges from the process of migraine. Migraine is aptly defined as a syndrome—a constellation of symptoms related to one another by physiologic peculiarity. An analysis of symptoms associated with migraine reveals that a wide array of physiologic dysfunctions can be observed during migraine. Symptom variations can be observed from patient to patient or between different attacks in the same patient, especially over the decades of headache activity before the patient finally seeks medical help.

The Spectrum Studies

Even in patients with migraine without aura diagnosed according to IHS criteria, there are often headache presentations that do not manifest sufficient symptomatology for migraine to be formally diagnosed. Some of these headaches are considered tension-type headache or migrainous headache, while others, perhaps with autonomic symptoms, may be improperly defined as "sinus headaches." The clinical observation is that migraineurs experience a variety of headache presentations. The question is: Do these different types of headaches represent different disorders with different pathophysiologies, or are they simply different points along a continuum of migraine evolution?

Raskin and others proposed that migraine and tension-type headache existed on a continuum of headache activity. Olesen later proposed that the phenotypic variability of migraine attacks can be explained by the integration of vascular, supraspinal, and myofascial inputs into the trigeminal system. This model provided insight into why muscle pain and other nonvascular symptoms often occur during migraine.

In 1997, Cady et al published a retrospective study of 1,904 treated attacks of migraine in a population of patients who, from clinical history and examination, had IHS migraine with or without aura. Enrollment in the study required a history of IHS migraine with or without aura. However, during the treatment phase of the study, investigators evaluated each attack of headache and recorded attack symptoms. Eligibility for treatment was based on the clinical diagnosis of migraine rather than IHS criteria. Each attack clinically diagnosed as migraine was treated with 6 mg subcutaneous sumatriptan.

Retrospective analysis of all treated headaches revealed that 43 patients had treated at least 1 headache that did not meet IHS criteria for migraine with or without aura. These non-IHS headaches met criteria for migrainous headache (meaning that they lacked 1 IHS criterion for migraine) or episodic tension-type headache (ETTH). Analysis of treatment response to 6 mg subcutaneous sumatriptan showed that all attack types responded equally well to treatment and, specifically, that pain relief was achieved by 95% for all attack types within 2 hours of treatment. Based on the consistency of response to sumatriptan, a treatment presumed to have specificity for migraine across all diagnostic categories, the authors suggested that the "spectrum" of primary headaches observed in established migraineurs shared common pathophysiologic mechanisms.

Lipton et al designed a prospective, randomized, placebo-controlled study to test these conclusions. The 454 subjects were divided into 3 groups based on their headache histories: migraine, migrainous, or ETTH. These subjects scored in the top 50% of individuals with migraine-related disability, as measured by the HIT. The subjects treated up to 10 headache attacks of moderate to severe pain with 50 mg sumatriptan or identical-appearing placebo with a randomization ratio of 4:1. Subjects kept detailed diaries and recorded symptoms that occurred during acute headaches.

Analysis of responses in the migraine group (ie, the subjects who experienced all 3 types of attacks) indicated that sumatriptan was superior to placebo in treating all headache presentations (migraine, migrainous, tension-type). These results confirmed those of the previous retrospective study that in migraineurs, the entire clinical spectrum of headaches may share a common underlying physiologic mechanism.

The treatment responses of the migrainous group (ie, subjects who had only migrainous and tension-type headache, but no migraine by strict IHS criteria) were also evaluated. Response to sumatriptan for this group revealed similar efficacy for migrainous and tension-type headache, and the responses were statistically superior to those with placebo. Further, the therapeutic response to sumatriptan in those with migrainous headache was similar to that recorded in the IHS-defined migraine group. This was the first time that the treatment response to a triptan had been studied prospectively in migrainous patients. The results suggest that a broader clinical definition of migraine may be appropriate.

In an analysis of retrospective Spectrum Study protocol violators, who did not wait to treat their headaches at moderate to severe intensity but instead treated the headaches earlier, when the pain was mild, a significant increase in the efficacy of sumatriptan was noted when headaches were treated during the mild headache phase of migraine compared to treatment during the moderate to severe headache phase. This observation has since been noted prospectively with both sumatriptan and other triptan medications, suggesting that the pathophysiologic process underlying the mild headache phase may be different or may be amenable to treatment compared to the pathophysiologic process generating moderate to severe headache. Burstein et al have done work on subjects at Beth Israel Hospital in Boston showing that treating migraine before the second-order neurons are recruited in the brain stem (central sensitization) favors higher triptan efficacy.

Ashina and colleagues reported calcitonin gene-related peptide (CGRP) levels (presumed to be specific for migraine) to be elevated when subjects diagnosed with tension-type headache reported their headaches to have a throbbing quality. It may be that CGRP is a biochemical marker for tension-type headache that is evolving into migrainous headache or migraine.

The Convergence Hypothesis

The Convergence Hypothesis proposes that migraine, migrainous, and tension-type headaches are not pathophysiologically distinct headache disorders, but are instead different phenotypic expressions of the same underlying physiologic process.

The Convergence Hypothesis suggests that the clinical expression of IHS migraine represents the full evolution of this pathophysiologic process and that tension-type and migrainous headache are clinical observations of the same process that has not evolved to its entirety (Figure, page 34). While further research needs to be done on this hypothesis, it is an attractive clinical model that explains the diversity of headache presentations seen in both an individual with migraine and the migraine population. The clinical foundation for this hypothesis is the Phase Model of migraine as proposed by Blau.

Phase Model of Migraine

An attack of migraine evolves over time through a predictable pattern. It can be divided into 3 general phases: preheadache, headache, and postheadache. Not all patients experience each phase, and not all patients display each migraine during the same phase. That is, some patients manifest no pre- or

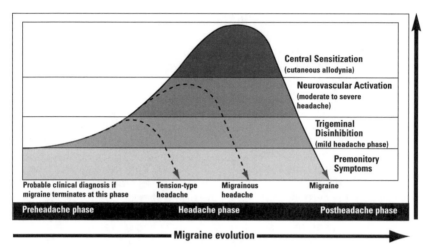

Figure. The convergence hypothesis.

postheadache phase, and some patients have a preheadache in some but not all attacks.

Preheadache Phase. Prodrome (premonitory symptoms) and aura constitute the preheadache phase. These are the earliest symptoms of the migraine process and can occur in advance of the headache. Prodromal symptoms include irritability, fatigue, food craving, cloudy thinking, mood swings, yawning, muscle tension, and fluid retention.

Auras, by contrast, are focal, reversible neurologic events. They are usually visual, such as scotomata, phonopsias (flashes), stars, spots, or bubbles within the entire visual field or one half of it, or halos around lights. Visual auras last about 20 to 30 minutes, often scintillate, may move across the visual field, and are usually followed by a headache in a variable period after the termination of the aura but within at most 60 minutes. Aura may also be somatosensory, such as tingling or numbness in the fingers, lips, or cheeks; it can also manifest as weakness, coordination problems, or speech dysfunction.

Approximately 70% of migraineurs report premonitory symptoms; 15% experience aura. In one study, 83% of individuals with prodromal symptoms predicted more than 50% of their attacks despite no formal education on the premonitory or prodromal phase of migraine. Equally important, however, is that not all prodromes or premonitory phases evolve into diagnosable migraine. Prodromes can occur and resolve without leading into headache. Likewise, an aura can occur without subsequent headache; this is termed *acephalgic migraine* or *migraine aura without headache.* These observations suggest that the physiologic process leading to migraine can be terminated without leading to IHS migraine. One study found that ingestion of naratriptan (Amerge) during prodrome appeared to prevent 60% of predicted migraine episodes. Other studies have suggested that antidopamine drugs (eg, metoclopramide) may be helpful in preventing migraine if taken during prodrome.

Headache Phase. The headache usually progresses from mild to moderate to severe pain. Early in the headache phase, when the pain is mild, the associated symptoms of nausea, photophobia, and phonophobia have usually not yet developed. Depending on the pattern of the headache, mild headache can last minutes to days. Headache sufferers often can continue to function without significant impairment. In most instances, activities are not proscribed by this phase of the migraine process.

On the other hand, the headache that is moderate to severe in intensity and accompanied by migraine-associated symptoms does produce significant impairment of function. This is the most studied phase of the migraine process, and the symptoms that occur during this phase serve as the basis for current diagnostic criteria. For a migraine to be diagnosed, the features include moderate to severe headache, often localized to one side, aggravated by activity, and associated with photophobia and phonophobia. Generally, this phase lasts 4 to 72 hours. Other common symptoms, but not necessary for diagnosis, range from osmophobia to blurred vision, nasal stuffiness, abdominal cramps, diarrhea, sweating, and pallor and muscle pain in the head and neck.

Postheadache Phase. Resolution of the headache and postdrome constitute the postheadache phase. The headache of migraine may resolve through sleep (not rest), effective medication, or vomiting, especially in children. Once the headache stops, there may be a "migraine hangover," similar to the symptoms encountered during the prodrome phase, such as fatigue, irritability, mood swings, and inability to eat. The postdrome can extend disability for 1 to 2 days.

Implications of the Convergence Model in Clinical Practice

The convergence model underscores the complexity of migraine and the fact that many symptoms may be observed during the clinical event of migraine. This model questions the rationale for elevating certain of these symptoms to diagnostic proportions while minimizing others, and suggests that much of the confusion over headache diagnosis is related to diagnostic models based on achieving certain symptoms. This is confounded further when clinicians encourage early intervention strategies (which have demonstrated improved treatment outcomes) rather than late treatment strategies (which rely on all diagnostic criteria being met before intervention is undertaken).

In a pragmatic sense, this lumping of treatments rather than splitting them encourages the physician to diagnose primary headache based on symptom interpretation, but in the context of the pattern of headache activity and its potential impact. Migrainous headache should be considered migraine. If associated muscle or autonomic symptoms are present, or osmophobia is observed rather than photophobia, a migraine diagnosis is still possible from the migrainous IHS criteria.

Conclusion

Migrainous headache is by IHS definition a category of migraine. It is a common presentation of migraine and, in many headache sufferers, the dominant presentation of migraine they experience. Unfortunately, it is often disguised as "sinus headache" or tension headache. Migrainous headache responds to treatment in a fashion similar to that for migraine without aura.

The value of understanding this presentation of migraine is that it broadens the diagnostic scope of headache and encourages providers to look beyond the stereotypical definitions of migraine that were modeled in clinical trials.

Editors' Note

Three chapters in this book—those by Drs. Kaniecki (page 18), Cady (page 27), and the editors (page 38)—deal with the spectrum of migraine as a variable presentation for patients. Dr. Cady points out that patients with tension-type, migrainous, and migraine presentations all respond to sumatriptan better than placebo, suggesting that they may all be points on what Raskin and others have referred to as the "continuum of benign recurring headache." Dr. Cady provides guidance on how to approach the spectrum in a patient: treat the migrainous headaches as migraine, and have the patient take the triptan early in the course of the headache to maximize outcome. Some migrainous headaches, with symptoms of sinus pain and nasal stuffiness, or of bilaterality and neck muscle involvement, are frequently misdiagnosed as sinus and tension-type headaches, respectively. Usually, these patients also respond to sumatriptan, as evidenced by previous studies, and, theoretically, to other triptans as well.

Diagnosis: Migrainous Headache

Selected Reading

Ashina M, Bendtsen L, Jensen R, et al. Plasma levels of calcitonin gene-related peptide in chronic tension-type headache. *Neurology.* 2000;55:1335-1339.

Blau JN. Adult migraine: the patient observed. In: Blau JN, ed. *Migraine: Clinical and Research Aspects.* Baltimore, Md: Johns Hopkins University Press; 1987:3-17.

Burstein R, Yarnitsky D. Goor-Aryeh I, Ransil BJ, Bajwa ZH. An association between migraine and cutaneous allodynia. *Ann Neurol.* 2000;47:614-624.

Cady RK, Gutterman D, Saiers JA, Beach ME. Responsiveness of non-IHS migraine and tension-type headache to sumatriptan. *Cephalalgia.* 1997;17:588-590.

Cady RK, Lipton RB, Hall C, et al. Treatment of mild headache in disabled migraine sufferers: results of the Spectrum Study. *Headache.* 2000;40:792-797.

Cady RK, Schreiber CP. Sinus or migraine? Considerations in making a differential diagnosis. *Neurology.* 2002;58(suppl 6):S10-S14.

Headache Classification Committee of the International Headache Society. Classification and diagnostic criteria for headache disorders, cranial neuralgias and facial pain. *Cephalalgia.* 1988;8(suppl 7):1-96.

International 311C90 Long-Term Study Group. The long-term tolerability and efficacy of oral zolmitriptan (Zomig, 311C90) in the acute treatment of migraine. *Headache.* 1998;38:173-183.

Kaniecki RG. Migraine and tension type headache: an assessment of challenges in diagnosis. *Neurology.* 2002;58(suppl 6):S15-S20.

Lipton RB, Stewart WF, Cady R, et al. Sumatriptan for the range of headaches in migraine sufferers: results of the Spectrum Study. *Headache.* 2000;40:783-791.

Lipton RB, Stewart WF, Diamond S, et al. Prevalence and burden of migraine in the United States: data from the American Migraine Study II. *Headache.* 2001;41:646-657.

Luciani R, Carter D, Mannix L, Hemphill M, Diamond M, Cady R. Prevention of migraine during prodrome with naratriptan. *Cephalalgia.* 2000;20:122-126.

Olesen J. Clinical and pathophysiological observations in migraine and tension-type headache explained by integration of vascular, supraspinal and myofascial inputs. *Pain.* 1991;46:125-132.

Pascual J, Falk R, Docekal R, et al. Tolerability and efficacy of almotriptan in the long-term treatment of migraine. *Eur Neurol.* 2001;45:206-213.

Raskin NH. *Headache.* 2nd ed. New York, NY: Churchill Livingstone; 1988.

Rozen TD, Swanson JW, Stang PE, McDonnell SK, Rocca WA. Increasing incidence of medically recognized migraine headache in a United States population. *Neurology.* 1999;53:1468-1473.

4. The Woman With a Spectrum of Headaches

Stewart J. Tepper, MD

Director, The New England Center for Headache
Stamford, Connecticut
Assistant Clinical Professor of Neurology
Yale University School of Medicine
New Haven, Connecticut

Alan M. Rapoport, MD

Director, The New England Center for Headache
Stamford, Connecticut
Clinical Professor of Neurology
Columbia University College of Physicians and Surgeons
New York, New York

Fred D. Sheftell, MD

Director, The New England Center for Headache
Stamford, Connecticut
Clinical Assistant Professor of Psychiatry
New York Medical College
Valhalla, New York

Case

ML is a 29-year-old right-handed woman who presented at our Headache Center with the chief complaint of worsening headache.

Her headaches had begun in childhood, but became more severe about 5 years ago. They occur in a spectrum: Headaches may be mild, moderate, or severe. She can't tell, at the beginning of any particular headache, how intense it will become.

ML never experiences a prodrome or aura. Headache onset occurs during the afternoon. The time to maximal intensity is 1 to 2 hours. The headaches are located posteriorly and anteriorly, including at the back of the head and neck, across the forehead, and into the temples. They are usually global or at least bilateral, but occasionally they are unilateral. The headaches can be steady, pressure-type pain, but at their worst, they are throbbing and associated with nausea, mild photophobia, and significant phonophobia. The pain is so intense at times that it prevents the performance of any activities, and the patient is confined to bed.

The moderate headaches are similar to the severe headaches, but "with the volume turned down," according to the patient. The moderate headaches occur without nausea, and with phonophobia but no photophobia.

The mild headaches are almost without distinguishing features. They occur without throbbing, nausea, photophobia, or phonophobia; unlike the moderate to severe headaches, they are not worsened by routine physical activity. The problem is that all of the patient's headaches begin this way.

The overall duration of her headaches is many hours, and they last for the remainder of the day. She then experiences a postdrome on the second day after a severe headache, consisting of a flu-like malaise during which she functions, but not up to capacity.

The frequency of attacks is about once a week for a mild to moderate headache, and up to twice monthly for the severe, disabling attacks. The headaches frequently occur on weekends, and so ML rarely misses work. However, when the patient experiences a moderate to severe headache on a weekday, she is unable to work.

Triggers for her headaches include fasting or delaying a meal, menses, stress, the letdown after stress, weekends, and dehydration. When the headaches occur with menstruation, they consistently begin on the first day of flow.

Occasionally, the mild and moderate headaches respond to naproxen sodium or butalbital combination medication, but the severe headaches never do. She has tried every over-the-counter (OTC) medication, without success. Her doctor has told her unequivocally that she does not have migraine, and the patient wonders about her diagnosis and the potential for treatment.

Allergies to Medication
None.

Current Medications
Levothyroxine sodium (Synthroid) 175 mcg, bupropion 100 mg qAM, nitrofurantoin prn, loratadine prn, naproxen sodium 550 mg prn (no more than 1 to 2 days of use per week), butalbital with acetaminophen 1 or 2 per day for headache prn (no more than 2 to 3 days of use per month), and aspirin/acetaminophen/diphenhydramine prn for sleep (never more than once or twice weekly).

Medical History
Positive for depression, anxiety, hypothyroidism, and recurrent tonsillitis.

Habits
The patient is a nonsmoker, drinks alcohol once or twice a week, has 1 caffeinated beverage per day, and uses no recreational drugs.

Surgical History
ML had bilateral myringotomies in childhood.

Family History
Her father has disabling migraine.

Social History
The patient is a teacher of special education. She is currently separated from her husband and under stress. They have no children. Her Migraine Disability Assessment Scale (MIDAS) score is only 5, but she describes the intensity of her attacks as ranging from 8 to 10 out of 10. Her Headache Impact Test (HIT)-6 score was 61, suggesting the very severe impact of headaches on her life.

Review of Systems

Positive for depression, anxiety, hypothyroidism, urethral and urinary tract infections, and low back pain; negative for seizures, trauma, diabetes, asthma, hypertension, heart murmur, heart disease, hypercholesterolemia, and glaucoma.

Exam

Blood pressure, 120/75; pulse, 72; and regular respiratory rate, 12. A general physical and detailed neurologic exam produced normal results except for a large asymmetric thyroid, left lobe greater than right, without masses.

Workup

Consisted of a computed tomographic scan of the head with contrast and also of the sinuses, both of which were normal, 1 year before consultation. A recent thyroid workup was negative.

Discussion

ML's severe headaches meet the International Headache Society (IHS) classification criteria for migraine without aura. The criteria that she meets are as follows:
1. Having had more than 5 attacks.
2. Headaches last from 4 hours to 72 hours (hers begin in the afternoon and are gone by the next morning).
3. Any 2 of the following 4 (ML has 3/4 [marked in italics]):
   a. *Moderate to severe intensity.*
   b. *Throbbing quality to the pain.*
   c. *Pain made worse with simple activity.*
   d. Unilateral location (ML's headaches are bilateral).
4. The headaches need to have either of the following (ML has both):
   a. Nausea and/or vomiting (she has nausea).
   b. Photophobia and/or phonophobia (she has both).
5. The patient needs to have a normal exam and/or imaging study.

Her moderate headaches either are moderate migraine by IHS criteria or meet the criteria for migrainous headache (see Cady chapter, page 27). Migrainous headaches meet all the IHS criteria for migraine except one. For example, the criteria require either nausea or both photophobia and phonophobia. The subject says that during her moderate attacks, she doesn't experience nausea, and gets phonophobia but not photophobia. Otherwise, the attacks are the same as the severe headaches but with only moderate intensity. Thus, some of her moderate attacks are migrainous, which is a migraine-type headache. Indeed, in 2002, the Food and Drug Administration stated that migrainous headache is a form of migraine.

Her mild headaches are phenotypically episodic tension-type headache (ETTH) (see Kaniecki chapter, page 18). They are featureless, without throbbing, and not worsened by routine physical activity, nausea, or photo- or phonophobia. The question thus becomes: Why don't these headaches always respond to naproxen sodium or butalbital mixtures?

The answer lies in understanding the spectrum of migraine. The key to this comes from the Spectrum Study (Lipton et al), which is described in the chapter by Dr. Cady, one of the study's authors. Before the Spectrum Study, there were 3 hypotheses as to the basis of these 3 types of headaches. The first was generated by Raskin and others in the 1980s. This hypothesis was that migraine and ETTH are the same disorder, differing in degree. At one end of the spectrum was migraine with aura, and at the other end, tension-type headache. Today, we could say that migrainous headaches fall in the middle. The major primary headaches occupy different ends of the same spectrum, which he called the "continuum of benign recurring headache."

The second hypothesis was actually included in the IHS classification system, and represents a view held widely in Europe, as described by Olesen. The European hypothesis is that migraine and ETTH are distinct disorders with independent biologic mechanisms. Presumably (although it is unproven), migrainous headache is migraine-type. Epidemiology actually suggests a difference between migraine and tension-type headache. Population studies have found that migraine is a disorder of lower socioeconomic class, while ETTH is linked to higher socioeconomic levels.

Finally, there is a third hypothesis, first put forward by Mathew and Sheftell, stating that there are really 2 types of ETTH:

ETTH in people with migraine may have "migraine-like" mechanisms (or may be low-level migraine at one end of the spectrum).

ETTH in people without migraine has a distinctly different mechanism. Clinically, we do see some patients with purely ETTH and, occasionally, even see the chronic form, but the first is not common and the second is also rare.

The Spectrum Study was laid out to distinguish between these hypotheses, based on response to triptans. Pharmacologic predictions were made on the basis of the 3 hypotheses:

1. If migraine headache, migrainous headaches, and ETTH are part of the same spectrum (the Raskin hypothesis), all 3 should respond equally well to triptans, and better than placebo.
2. If migraine headache, migrainous headache, and ETTH are biologically distinct (the European hypothesis), then only migraine, and not ETTH, should respond to triptans. If migrainous headache is a type of migraine, it should respond as migraine.
3. If the third hypothesis is correct, ETTH in people with migraine should respond to triptans, because migraine patients have a full spectrum in their presentation of migraine; ETTH in people without migraine should not respond to triptans better than placebo.

Thus, the Spectrum Study can be set up as a matrix:

Attack Presentations			
Patient type 1	Migraine	Migrainous	ETTH
Patient type 2		Migrainous	ETTH
Patient type 3			ETTH

A line would be drawn horizontally between patient types 2 and 3. The third type of patient, those with "pure" tension-type headache, would not respond to triptans, while all those above the line, regardless of the presentation of their attacks, would respond to triptans, as all of their attacks are migraine variants.

It turned out to be very hard to find a patient with pure, disabling ETTH, because at least one third of the patients recruited into the study with that diagnosis turned out to have migraine or migrainous headache, as evidenced by analysis of the diaries of their attacks collected over the length of the study. However, even allowing for the smaller group of subjects in the study who turned out to be true type 3 patients (pure ETTH), the Sheftell/Mathew hypothesis turned out to be correct.

All patients in the study received either sumatriptan 50 mg tablets or placebo for up to 10 attacks over 6 months. Placebo was given for 20% of attacks. The results were that sumatriptan successfully treated patients with migraine, migrainous headaches, and ETTH, when the 3 headaches or 2 out of 3 were attack types occurring in the same subjects over time. However, there was no difference in response to sumatriptan vs placebo in the pure ETTH patients.

There are 2 types of ETTH: the type that occurs in a spectrum with migraine and migrainous headaches in the same patient (probably just low-level migraine) and the type that occurs in isolation. What is seen in the office when a patient complains of headache is almost always migraine and the spectrum of migraine. This has become appreciated in the Landmark Study, presented at several meetings in 2002 but available only in abstract form at the time of the printing of this book.

The Landmark Study set out to determine what type of headache patients actually complained of in primary care offices (based on IHS criteria) throughout the world. This was a prospective, open-label, multicenter, international study of primary care physicians from 14 countries and 128 centers. A patient was eligible for inclusion in the study if he or she complained of headache (not necessarily as the chief complaint); 1,217 individuals were enrolled. Each patient reported his or her own diagnosis and was also given a diagnosis by a primary care physician. Patients with migraine or non-migraine headache newly diagnosed by their primary care physicians were given diaries to record up to 6 attacks. Each attack was then reviewed by an expert panel, and assigned a diagnosis based on IHS criteria. A final diagnosis was given for each patient based on the worst attack.

The results were fascinating, and confirm the spectrum of migraine. First, when the primary care physician diagnosed a migraine, the diagnosis was correct by IHS criteria 98% of the time for a migraine-type headache (migraine and migrainous). If a patient self-diagnosed migraine, the patient was correct by IHS criteria for a migraine-type headache in 99.5% of cases. However, if the primary care doctor diagnosed a nonmigraine headache, the likelihood was that the diagnosis was wrong. Eighty-two percent of these patients had migraine-type headache. If the patient self-diagnosed nonmigraine headache, the likelihood was that that the diagnosis was wrong as well, as 87% of these patients had migraine-type headache.

The pattern of the attacks in the patients who received a diagnosis of migraine was different over 6 attacks from those in patients who received an incorrect, nonmigraine diagnosis. The patients who received a migraine diagnosis experienced 73% of their attacks as pure migraine by IHS criteria, 23% of their attacks as migrainous, and only 4% of their attacks as ETTH. The patients who received an incorrect diagnosis of nonmigraine, on the other hand, experienced 36% of their attacks as pure migraine, 47% as migrainous, and 17% as tension-type.

Thus, the end of the spectrum at which a patient's attacks cluster can both affect the patient's own perception of the nature of the headaches and alter the doctor's diagnosis. Most of these patients had migraine, regardless of the misdiagnosis, so many did not receive optimal treatment.

Patients with disabling attacks of migraine, regardless of the presentation, merit migraine-specific treatment (ie, with triptans) and will do better if they receive triptan therapy at the start of their acute attacks. The evidence for this can be seen in the Disabilities in Strategies of Care (DISC) study. In this study, Lipton et al addressed 3 strategies for treating patients with disabling attacks of migraine: step care across attacks, step care within attacks, and stratified care.

Step care across attacks involves starting patients with a low-level, nonspecific treatment for migraines, regardless of whether the attacks are disabling, and switching to a triptan only if the lower-level treatments fail after being tried for several attacks. That strategy wastes time, and can cause discomfort, pain, and disability for each poorly treated attack.

Step care within attacks is the strategy of initially treating with a nonspecific medication and using a triptan only if the headache does not respond if the attack progresses despite the nonspecific treatment. With this strategy, triptans are used as rescue medications, and are often given so late in the attack that there is less of a chance of a good response. The patient also loses time and endures pain and disability until the triptan works.

Stratified care is defined as initially matching a patient's or an attack's characteristics to the appropriate treatment. Lipton and Stewart's contribution to the concept of stratified care was to suggest that the patient's disability, the impact on the patient's life, and/or the time loss from headache could be used as a surrogate marker for disease severity. Their idea was to use a disability measuring tool (MIDAS) to gauge disability and then to stratify treatment to triptans (zolmitriptan in the study) for moderately to severely disabled patients, while administering nonspecific treatment (aspirin and metoclopramide) to the less severely disabled patients.

All parameters of patient outcome were better for the stratified group in the DISC study. Post hoc analysis has shown that stratified care was also less expensive. What this means clinically is that asking about time lost from normal life because of headache is an excellent strategy for selecting appropriate acute care treatment for the patient with episodic migraine, and allows initial implementation of a correct treatment plan. Patients with greater time loss, impact, or disability, as measured by any of the validated tools available (eg, MIDAS, HIT), should be given a triptan for their attacks.

Treatment

The patient in this case had the spectrum of migraine, and experienced disabling attacks at least once or twice a week. The treatment was a 100-mg sumatriptan tablet given in the mild phase of headache and repeated in 2 hours in the rare case it was needed. If the patient awoke with a full-blown headache or needed faster relief, 6 mg sumatriptan was given by subcutaneous self-injection. This treatment strategy generally worked in 20 minutes, removing both the pain and the associated symptoms.

Conclusion

The key to understanding migraine is realizing that it presents in different ways in the same person, as well as from patient to patient. The term "spectrum of migraine" means that patients with disabling migraine may present with attacks that meet IHS criteria for migraine, migrainous headache, or even episodic tension-type headache. Each of these attacks should respond to a triptan.

We know from the DISC study that patients with disabling attacks should be given triptans for their attacks as a first-line strategy, and that outcomes will be better, and costs lower.

From the Landmark Study, it is now clear that the vast majority of patients complaining of headache in the primary care office have migraine. (Patients with pure tension-type headache usually do not have the pain intensity or disability of the migraineurs and rarely complain to their doctors about headache.) If migraine patients begin to overuse analgesics and develop rebound headaches, they might complain about increasing frequency and intensity of headache, gastrointestinal problems, or easy bruising.

The key is to recognize the spectrum of the attacks in a migraineur. Most patients complaining of headache have migraine, experience significant impact from their headaches, and have disability or time loss. In these cases, individuals should be given triptans as the first-line medication.

Diagnosis: Migraine, Migrainous, and Episodic Tension-Type Headache in the Same Patient: The Full Spectrum of Migraine

Selected Reading

Dowson A, Tepper SJ, Newman L, Dahlof C. The prevalence and diagnosis of migraine in a primary care setting: insights from the Landmark Study. *Cephalalgia*. 2002;22:590-591.

Headache Classification Committee of the International Headache Society. Classification and diagnostic criteria for headache disorders, cranial neuralgias and facial pain. *Cephalalgia*. 1988;8(suppl 7):1-96.

Lipton RB, Stewart WF, Cady R, et al. Sumatriptan for the range of headaches in migraine sufferers: results of the Spectrum Study. *Headache*. 2000;40:783-791.

Lipton RB, Stewart WF, Stone AM, et al. Stratified care vs. step care strategies for migraine. The Disability in Strategies of Care (DISC) Study. *JAMA*. 2000;284:2599-2605.

Raskin NH, ed. *Headache*. 2nd ed. New York, NY: Churchill Livingstone; 1988.

5. Sinus Headache:
A Case of Mistaken Identity

David W. Dodick, MD, FRCP, FACP

Associate Professor of Neurology
Mayo Medical School
Rochester, Minnesota
Consultant
Department of Neurology
Mayo Clinic
Scottsdale, Arizona

Case

A 48-year-old retired male police officer was referred for headache subspecialty consultation for disabling and recurrent sinus headaches, which were resistant to medical and surgical therapy.

His headaches began at age 8 years and have continued in an intermittent pattern. The character has remained relatively consistent, but the frequency of headache attacks and the severity of each have increased over the past 10 years.

At the time of consultation, diary records revealed an attack frequency of approximately 4 per month, each lasting approximately 72 hours. The headaches were typically unilateral and frontal, but attacks would alternate sides. The pain intensity was invariably severe, throbbing, and/or pressured.

Each attack was associated with nausea but rarely emesis. There was no associated photophobia or phonophobia, but each attack was either preceded (30 to 60 minutes) or associated with ipsilateral nasal congestion and tearing (lacrimation). His ability to function was severely limited, and during headaches he felt best in a reclining position.

Movement aggravated his headache. He had identified weather changes (especially barometric pressure/humidity changes during monsoon season), high altitude, aged cheese, and alcoholic beverages as relatively consistent triggers for headache.

Exam

General physical and neurologic examination gave normal results.

Past Medical History, Surgical History, and Hospitalizations

The patient had been diagnosed with recurrent "sinus headache." He underwent debridement of the left frontal and maxillary sinus and bilateral middle turbinectomies in 1989. Unfortunately, this did not reduce the frequency or intensity of his headaches, and he has had recurrent epistaxis since this procedure.

He had also been treated with an intraoral appliance for temporomandibular dysfunction, desensitization injections for several allergens, and several nasal decongestants and steroids.

He had received numerous courses of oral antibiotics for presumed recurrent sinusitis. Unfortunately, because none of these treatments provided relief, he experienced an upper gastrointestinal hemorrhage related to nonsteroidal anti-inflammatory drug–induced peptic ulcer disease as a result of using in excess of 3 g aspirin per day for each headache.

Laboratory and Imaging Workup

The patient's most recent imaging study was a magnetic resonance imaging scan of the brain and a computed tomography scan of the paranasal sinuses, which revealed mild mucosal edema in the left frontal and maxillary sinuses. This was interpreted as probably reflecting postoperative changes.

Discussion and Treatment

This patient is finally diagnosed with migraine without aura, and treated with an oral triptan for acute symptomatic relief. He achieves an excellent response, experiencing complete headache relief within 90 minutes of triptan administration. Because of his excellent and consistent response to acute symptomatic medication, the subject declines the offer of migraine preventive therapy.

Recent epidemiologic studies show that migraine is an extremely common and often debilitating neurologic disorder in the United States, affecting approximately 18% of women and 6% of men. The mean frequency of migraine headaches has been estimated to be approximately 1 to 2 per month, with headache severity characterized as "severe" or "very severe" by 60% to 80% of migraine sufferers in the general population. Overall, the World Health Organization ranks migraine among the world's most disabling medical illnesses.

Despite the frequency, severity, and negative economic and functional impact of migraine on quality of life, some recent surveys suggest that less than half of current migraineurs have ever received a medical diagnosis. Consistent with this, International Medical Statistics audit data suggest that in the year 2000, only 17% of migraineurs were receiving treatment with prescription drugs.

Even though healthcare utilization has increased among migraineurs, only 50% to 71% of patients who have consulted a physician for migraine have received the diagnosis. While the reasons for this may be multifactorial, even under ideal circumstances, appropriate diagnosis may be difficult. Any individual IHS criterion symptom of migraine, such as nausea, photophobia, or phonophobia, may be absent in as many as 40% of migraine sufferers. Furthermore, physicians may rely on aura for diagnosis, a feature that is absent in more than two-thirds of migraine sufferers.

If these patients are not receiving a diagnosis of migraine, what diagnosis are they given? A recent epidemiologic study revealed that of the patients who met the International Headache Society (IHS) criteria for migraine but received a different diagnosis, 42% received a diagnosis of sinus headache.

In a recent study of 37 patients who were referred with either a self-diagnosis or physician diagnosis of sinus headache, 36/37 (98%) were found to have migrainous (11/37) or migraine (25/37) headache after application of the IHS diagnostic criteria. Furthermore, the 2-hour headache response rate to sumatriptan 50 mg was 63% and 68%, respectively, when these 2 groups of patients treated a moderate or severe headache.

In another study, involving 2,524 patients who presented to their physician with either a self-described or physician-diagnosed sinus headache, 62% (1,560) fulfilled IHS criteria for migraine without aura; 20%, migraine with aura; and 8%, migrainous headache. In addition to typical migraine symptoms (photophobia, nausea), patients frequently reported symptoms that are often associated with sinus disease, such as nasal congestion, rhinorrhea, tearing (lacrimation), and pressure over the frontal or maxillary facial region. Furthermore, 84% of these patients reported substantial headache-related disability and dissatisfaction (66%) with their acute symptomatic therapy.

The presence of cranial autonomic symptoms such as tearing, nasal congestion, and rhinorrhea during migraine attacks is not surprising. In a recent study of 177 consecutive migraine sufferers, ipsilateral autonomic symptoms were reported by 81 patients (45.8%); ocular symptoms alone or in combination with nasal symptoms were the most frequent. The headache was more severe and more strictly unilateral in patients who reported these symptoms than in those without.

Why is migraine so often mistaken for sinus headache? There are likely several reasons for these cases of mistaken identity. First and foremost, symptoms traditionally associated with allergic rhinitis or rhinosinusitis, as described above, commonly occur during migraine attacks. This is not entirely surprising, given the innervation of the nasal and sinus mucosa and the underlying pathophysiology of migraine.

Sensory, parasympathetic, and sympathetic nerves regulate epithelial, vascular, glandular, and smooth muscle functions that affect the nasal and pharyngeal mucosa, protecting these airways from injury caused by inhaled irritants and infection. They also participate in the pathogenesis of allergic and nonallergic rhinitis and asthma. The nasal sensory nerves originate in the trigeminal ganglion and innervate the nasal and sinus mucosa by means of branches of the first and second divisions of the trigeminal nerve.

Nociceptive (pain) fibers are stimulated by inflammatory mediators involved in rhinitis. Afferent (feedback, retrograde) activation of the trigeminal sensory (nociceptive) system by inflammation within the paranasal or nasal mucosa could thus trigger migraine by affecting the brain stem in a susceptible individual.

Similarly, activation of the cranial parasympathetic system, which provides vasomotor innervation to the cerebral blood vessels and secretomotor innervation to the nasal and sinus mucosa and lacrimal glands, explains why patients with cluster headache and chronic paroxysmal hemicrania experience robust cranial autonomic symptoms such as tearing, nasal congestion, and rhinorrhea during attacks. This system has been shown to be activated during migraine attacks in patients who also develop these autonomic symptoms in measurements of significantly elevated levels of vasoactive intestinal polypeptide (a parasympathetic neurotransmitter) in the jugular venous blood during attacks of migraine. Activation of this normal human anatomic pathway is the likely mechanism by which sinus-like symptoms are seen so often during acute migraine attacks.

A second reason for the confusion between sinus headache and migraine is the location of pain during acute attacks of migraine. Migraine is, of course, a referred pain syndrome. The first division (ophthalmic) of the trigeminal nerve conveys much of the nociceptive information from pain-sensitive intracranial contents (including the dura mater and cerebral blood vessels), while the second (maxillary) transmits nociceptive information from the contents of the middle cranial fossa. Referred pain can also be sent down these pathways, making the patient feel the pain in the sinus regions. Thus, it is no surprise that headache pain is often felt in the frontal and sometimes in the maxillary regions—the very areas that overlie the paranasal sinuses that are the most frequently involved with allergic rhinitis and rhinosinusitis.

Furthermore, some of the most common migraine triggers are weather pattern changes (barometric pressure, humidity), high altitude, perfumes, cigarette smoke, and other irritant odors. It is, therefore, not entirely surprising that the patient described above, with acute, recurrent, unilateral frontal headaches triggered by weather changes and altitude, and associated with nasal congestion and rhinorrhea, received a diagnosis of "sinus headache" regardless of the other typical migraine symptoms (eg, nausea) that were present.

Another cause for confusion is the prevalence of "pathologic findings" on sinus radiographic studies. In a large study involving 666 asymptomatic subjects who underwent sinus scans, mucosal thickening, polyps, or opacification in one or more sinus cavities was found in 42% of this population. In patients with primary headache disorders such as migraine or cluster headache, because of the frequent clinical involvement of the nasal and sinus mucosa as described, mucosal thickening or opacification has been demonstrated in sinus radiographs in as many as 96% of patients, in the absence of rhinosinusitis.

Rhinosinusitis

Because of the overlapping clinical features, the distinction between acute rhinosinusitis and migraine is clearly important. The American Academy of Otolaryngology–Head and Neck Surgery developed a consensus opinion on working definitions of acute, subacute, and chronic rhinosinusitis. They concluded that thorough history and physical examination are sufficient for the routine diagnosis of most forms of rhinosinusitis.

The examination should include anterior rhinoscopy, otoscopy, and oropharyngeal and neck examinations. They identified major and minor clinical symptoms and signs believed to be most significant for accurate clinical diagnosis of all forms of adult rhinosinusitis (Table 1, page 50).

Clinical findings consistent with rhinosinusitis must include 2 or more major factors or 1 major and 2 minor factors. While facial pain and pressure are major symptoms, headache is considered a minor symptom. Similarly, the revised criteria proposed by the IHS required simultaneous onset of headache and rhinosinusitis, the latter of which is documented clinically or by imaging studies (Table 2, page 50).

The temporal pattern of migraine is perhaps the single feature that best distinguishes this syndrome from acute sinusitis. In the American Migraine

Study II, 25% of women who have migraine experience 4 or more severe attacks per month; 35% experience 1 to 4 severe attacks per month; and 38% experience 1 or no severe attacks per month. In the same study, 92% of women and 89% of men with severe migraine had some headache-related disability. About half were severely disabled or needed bed rest.

Furthermore, migraine attacks tend to be stereotyped within individuals with relatively consistent triggers (menstruation, stress, sleep deprivation, etc). This relatively frequent, repetitive, and stereotyped pattern is generally not seen in patients with acute sinusitis. The patient described reported the onset of his headaches as having occurred when he was 8 years old. The headaches were stereotyped, and never changed significantly in character, but became more frequent and severe. Given this history, a diagnosis of recurrent sinusitis over 40 years is implausible.

Whether headache can be seen as a feature of recurrent allergic or nonallergic rhinitis is unclear. Because individual migraine sufferers often have more than 1 headache type, it is possible that nasal or sinus inflammation in these patients can trigger a migraine, a migrainous headache, or headache with an entirely different phenotype. This is an area that clearly needs further study. Certainly, intermittent mucosal inflammation and edema may lead to mucosal contact point headache, an entity now recognized by the IHS (Table 3, page 51).

A careful clinical history of different headache types is thus important for patients with migraine. If there is suspicion of mucosal contact point headache, appropriate imaging studies are recommended. Other diseases, such as deviated nasal septum, hypertrophic turbinate, atrophic sinus membranes, and chronic sinusitis, are entities that, according to the IHS, are not sufficiently validated as a cause of facial pain or headache.

Conclusion

Migraine is often mistakenly diagnosed as "sinus headache" or true acute rhinosinusitis, in large part because of the location of pain and associated sinus-like symptoms. The pain of migraine frequently overlies the paranasal sinuses—particularly the frontal sinus.

There is a group of migraine patients who, in addition to fulfilling the criteria for migraine without aura, may have clinical features such as facial (maxillary) pain, nasal congestion, rhinorrhea, and tearing. These patients do not have mucopurulent nasal discharge or other abnormalities seen in acute rhinosinusitis. Therefore, it is necessary to differentiate rhinosinusitis-causing headache from what has been referred to as "sinus headaches"—which are generally headache attacks fulfilling the IHS criteria for migraine without aura—from nasal symptoms due to concomitant mucosal edema.

Coexistent nasal or sinus symptoms may occur as a result of parasympathetic activation during migraine or, possibly, migraine that is triggered by inflammatory mucosal changes due to noninfectious rhinitis. Whether headache can be seen with allergic or nonallergic rhinitis has not been clearly answered, and whether migraine sufferers are more susceptible to non-migraine headaches triggered by nasal or sinus mucosal inflammation, acute sinusitis, or septal contact point headache is an area in need of further study.

Table 1. Major and Minor Factors for the Diagnosis of Rhinosinusitis

Major factors

- Facial pain/pressure/congestion/fullness
- Fever (in acute rhinosinusitis only)
- Hyposmia/anosmia
- Nasal obstruction/blockage/discharge/purulence
- Purulence in nasal cavity on examination

Minor factors

- Cough
- Dental pain
- Ear pain/pressure/fullness
- Fatigue
- Fever
- Halitosis
- Headache

Editors' Note

Dr. Dodick describes a type of patient seen all too often in a headache practice: one with migraine without aura who experiences vasomotor instability with migraine attacks, and who is misdiagnosed as having "sinus headache" and mistreated with antibiotics, antihistamines, decongestants, and, in this case, ultimately harmful or unhelpful and unnecessary surgery. There is reason to question the existence of a separate entity called "sinus headache."

While headache is a secondary feature of sinusitis, the syndrome of recurrent, stereotypical episodes of infectious sinusitis/headache triggered after stress or at menses is not clinically validated. The SUMMIT study, presented at the American Headache Society meeting in Seattle, of more than 2,500 people with "sinus headache" found that more than 90% met IHS criteria for migraine-type headache.

It is likely that "sinus headache" is an American invention of advertising for OTC antihistamines and decongestants. Indeed, the diagnostic entity of "sinus headache" does not exist in Europe and is not included in the IHS clas-

Table 2. International Headache Society Criteria for Acute Rhinosinusitis Headache

- Pain perceived in 1 or more regions of the head, face, ears, or teeth
- Clinical, laboratory, and/or imaging evidence of an acute rhinosinusitis—eg, purulence in nasal cavity, nasal obstruction, fever, hyposmia/anosmia, CT imaging, MR imaging, or fiber-optic endoscopy findings
- Simultaneous onset of headache and rhinosinusitis
- Headache disappears after remission of the acute rhinosinusitis

CT, computed tomography; MR, magnetic resonance

Table 3. International Headache Society Criteria for Mucosal Contact Point Headache

- Intermittent pain localized to the periorbital and medial canthal or temporozygomatic regions
- Clinical and/or imaging evidence of mucosal contact points by nasal endoscopy of CT imaging and no findings of acute rhinosinusitis
- Evidence that the pain can be attributed to mucosal contact point, based on at least 1 of the following 3 criteria:

  1. Headache is corresponding to variations in mucosal congestion mediated by gravitational changes when the patient is vertical or horizontal

  2. Abolition of headache within 30 seconds after topical application of cocaine to the middle turbinate using placebo or other controls

  3. Headache disappears after removal of mucosal contact points

CT, computed tomography

sification system that has been adopted by American professional journals and organizations.

Thus, when a patient informs the primary care physician or neurologist of a history of "sinus headache," skepticism and a low threshold for a migraine diagnosis seem in order.

Diagnosis: Migraine Without Aura Masquerading as "Sinus Headache"

Selected Reading

Blumenthal HJ. Headaches and sinus disease. *Headache.* 2001;41:883-888.

Cady RK, Schreiber CP. Sinus headache or migraine: considerations in making a differential diagnosis. *Neurology.* 2002;58(suppl 6):S10-S14.

International Headache Society Classification Criteria: Revised Edition, 2002 [www.i-h-s.org]

Lanza DC, Kennedy DW. Adult rhinosinusitis defined. *Otolaryngol Head Neck Surg.* 1997;117:S1-S7.

Lipton RB, Diamond S, Reed M, Diamond ML, Stewart WF. Migraine diagnosis and treatment: results from the American Migraine Study II. *Headache.* 2001;41:638-645.

6. The Woman With Frequent Headaches And Medication Use

Sylvia Lucas, MD, PhD

Co-director, Headache and MS Center, Swedish Neuroscience Institute
Clinical Assistant Professor of Neurology
University of Washington School of Medicine
Seattle, Washington

Case

A 52-year-old woman was referred by her headache specialist for management of her chronic and severe headache problem. She had been on disability for migraine headaches for approximately 5 years.

Her headaches had begun at age 20, and were severe 2 to 3 times a month, lasting up to 4 days. The headaches began in the left supraorbital area, spreading to the whole left side; they were throbbing and were accompanied by nausea, vomiting, and rhinorrhea. She would miss work approximately 2 days per month. Strong smells such as those of cigarette smoke and perfume, as well as alcohol and dairy products, were identifiable migraine triggers.

Past Medical History

Significant for anxiety disorder and peptic ulcer disease.

Family History

Included a father with paranoid schizophrenia.

Diagnostic Evaluation

By age 40, this patient's workup had included normal brain magnetic resonance imaging, electroencephalogram, plain sinus X-rays, and an ENT evaluation.

Past Medicines History and Disease Course

Preventive therapies had included the long-acting ergot preparations, ß-blockers, and tricyclics, which were all relatively ineffective. Acute therapies included aspirin, diazepam, butalbital compounds, propoxyphene, acetaminophen with codeine, oxycodone, and naproxen sodium, none of which were dramatically effective.

By age 42, she was waking up with headache and taking 6 to 12 aspirin tablets daily to keep her headache intensity to 2 on a 10-point scale. She also began taking butalbital–acetaminophen–caffeine with codeine, averaging 6 to 12 capsules daily.

Finally, at age 47, she was admitted to an inpatient headache center for 4 weeks, but still had daily headaches at discharge. Very soon after discharge, she began taking sumatriptan (Imitrex) daily.

The subject then underwent a second detoxification attempt at her local hospital to eliminate the daily sumatriptan, but the best she had ever done was 2 days a month without headache. By that time, preventive therapy had also included calcium channel blockers, valproic acid (Depakote), gabapentin (Neurontin), riboflavin, and magnesium.

At age 52, her daily pattern was to set her alarm for 6 AM and wake up to see whether she had a headache. She would wake with a headache 80% of the time; even if it was mild, she would take sumatriptan or rizatriptan (Maxalt) and go back to sleep. She would generally wake up headache-free at 8 AM, but headache would recur by midafternoon. She would take a second triptan tablet and/or aspirin at that time.

The 20% of the time she did not have a headache at 6 AM, it would occur by midmorning. The subject was using at least 30 rizatriptan and sumatriptan tablets per month.

She was hospitalized a third time for detoxification from rizatriptan and sumatriptan. The subject administered her last triptan on the morning of admission and was started immediately on intravenous dihydroergotamine (D.H.E. 45) q8 hours. She responded quickly to dihydroergotamine and became headache-free within 3 days.

At variable times during her hospitalization, the subject experienced anxiety, diarrhea, and nausea. Laboratory work produced normal results, with the exception of mild hypothyroidism, and she was started on levothyroxine. She began preventive therapy with long-acting venlafaxine (Effexor), citalopram (Celexa), and amitriptyline.

During her hospitalization, the subject was seen by a physical therapist for biofeedback and by a cognitive behavioral psychologist, who identified important negative behavior patterns. One such pattern was taking medication in anticipation of pain. Fear of pain would cause her to take medication prophylactically even if she were just going to participate in an event that she was "sure" would bring on a headache. Her failure to follow recommended therapy would then result in self-punishment with poor dietary habits, catastrophic thinking, and anxiety about the future. She could not distinguish her anxiety from her migraine headaches.

After 1 year of weekly therapy sessions that gradually decreased in frequency, and completion of an 8-week wellness program, she was able to control her migraines with triptan use 2 or 3 days per week. She learned pain and stress management strategies and, at onset of pain, developed insight into maladaptive responses that increased and sustained pain, versus responses that decreased pain. On occasion, she recognized the re-emergence of negative behavior patterns and returned to her psychologist. Following this regimen, she has done well for the past 2 years.

Discussion

Patients with frequent headache often overuse medication to prevent escalation of pain and to be able to function. In patients with primary headache disorders, months or years of frequent medication overuse can produce "rebound headache."

Rebound headache has been defined as "a self-sustaining, rhythmic headache medication cycle characterized by daily or near-daily headache and irresistible and predictable use of immediate relief medications as the only means of relieving headache attacks" (Saper and Jones, 1986). This case illustrates several characteristics of rebound headache, but also some of the inherent difficulties in dealing with these patients. They often have had years of medication overuse, in addition to psychiatric comorbidities and maladaptive behavior patterns that may be much more difficult to deal with than the relatively simple detoxification from overused medication.

The term "transformed migraine" was introduced by Mathew et al (1987) to describe daily or near-daily headache that in tertiary care centers can constitute 70% to 80% of the chronic daily headache population. Typically, these patients have a history of episodic migraine, with or without aura, starting in their teens or 20s.

Transformation from episodic to daily headache is usually gradual, although sudden transformation may be seen, particularly after head and neck trauma or medical illness. Clinical features of the headache may change as well, and can provide a clue that transformation has taken place. A chronic low-grade headache, indistinguishable from tension-type headache, often appears that is usually global or bilateral and typically involves the neck or occiput.

There are episodes of the patients' prior migraine headache type occurring every few days or weeks within this daily pattern. Headaches can be accompanied by asthenia, nausea, restlessness, anxiety or depression, irritability, nonrestorative sleep disorder, and difficulty with memory and concentration. Many of these symptoms are a consequence of the medication's having been overused. For example, chronic opiate use can produce a syndrome of depression, anxiety, memory difficulties, and mild withdrawal symptoms between doses (eg, restlessness, inability to sleep, nausea, irritability).

Perhaps the most characteristic feature of drug-dependent rebound headache is its early-morning periodicity. In this patient, headache was always present in the morning, mostly occurring before she woke up at 6 AM and always by midmorning. Usually the headaches are a withdrawal effect from the previous day's dose, but timing of the headache recurrence is not always predictable. The half-life of the medication, the timing of the last dose before sleep, the quantity of medication, and concomitant drug use can all vary the recurrence, but they tend to be consistent for each patient if drug use is unchanged.

Although rebound has not been studied in placebo-controlled trials, one study of caffeine discontinuation illustrates "withdrawal." In a double-blind, placebo-controlled trial (Silverman et al, 1992), 64 adults with low to moderate caffeine intake (approximately 2.5 cups per day) were given placebo or replacement caffeine during a 2-day caffeine-free controlled diet. By day 2, 50% of the patients given placebo versus 6% of those given caffeine had headache. Nausea, depression, and flu-like symptoms were common in the placebo group.

Withdrawal symptoms are also seen if overused medication is discontinued abruptly, usually accompanied by an increase in headache intensity and frequency. Other symptoms of withdrawal depend, of course, on the type and quantity of symptomatic medication consumed.

A sudden withdrawal of large quantities of barbiturates or benzodiazepines may put a patient at risk for withdrawal seizures. In many cases, a carefully orchestrated taper is medically necessary and possibly requires hospitalization. Dosing intervals may be critical enough with frequent drug use, and withdrawal symptoms so unpleasant that patients will carry the medication with them at all times, reinforcing a psychological as well as a physical dependence on "the only medicine that helps my headaches."

Another feature of rebound headache is development of drug tolerance. Initially, symptomatic medication may give relief with lower and less-frequent dosing. But as use increases, patients use larger quantities more frequently to provide the same—and in many cases incomplete—pain relief.

Of 200 chronic headache patients studied by Mathew et al (1990), 35% were using only 1 medication, but 43% were using 2 concomitantly and 22% were using 3 or more. In that series, the most frequent symptomatic medication used by 42% of the patients was butalbital–aspirin or acetaminophen–caffeine with or without codeine, with an average use of 30 tablets per week. Preparations also included other codeine-containing medications, used by 40% (average, 28 tablets per week), aspirin–acetaminophen–caffeine by 25% (average, 42 tablets per week), followed by ergotamine preparations, simple analgesics, codeine derivatives, decongestants, and antihistamines.

Actual drug dosages and the time necessary to develop drug-induced rebound have not been established. There may be large individual differences in susceptibility to rebound, and factors such as psychiatric comorbidity, the class of medication and its pharmacokinetic properties, and number of medications used may all play a part. Patterns of medication use predict rebound in patients who take 3 or more simple analgesics per day on more than 5 days per week; triptans or combination analgesics containing barbiturates, opiates, or caffeine more than 3 days per week; or opioids or ergotamine preparations more than 2 days per week (Silberstein and Lipton, 2001).

It has also been observed that patients likely to develop rebound are those who have primary headache disorders. Patients without headache history who take chronic analgesics for other conditions (eg, osteoarthritis) are unlikely to develop rebound, while those with episodic migraine histories who take analgesics for other conditions may develop daily headache. Similarly, rebound can also occur if a patient begins using analgesics again after detoxification for a condition other than headache.

Virtually any symptomatic medication used to treat headache can cause rebound, and substances used for other conditions (such as decongestants or antihistamines in cold preparations) or the consumption of caffeine in coffee, tea, colas, or other sodas may be suspect. Prolonged use of large quantities of aspirin, acetaminophen, or nonsteroidal anti-inflammatory drugs may have adverse effects on liver and kidney function, besides causing rebound headache.

Treatment

In a series of drug-induced refractory headaches, Mathew et al (1990) found that of 116 patients who were on concomitant prophylactic medications in addition to overused symptomatic medications, all experienced daily or near-daily headaches. Unless patients with rebound are willing to stop the use of such symptomatic medications, there is little chance that their headaches will resolve purely in response to the addition of one or more prophylactic agents.

However, discontinuation of the medication causing rebound will typically relieve the headache. Research (Diener et al, 1993) has shown that abrupt withdrawal of analgesics without other treatment but antiemetics, while causing short-term intense headache and withdrawal symptoms, results in a significant percentage of patients being headache-free or in large reductions in headache frequency over time.

Another important characteristic of rebound is the lack of response to preventive or migraine-specific medications during the overuse period. Detoxification restores the effectiveness of preventive medication and triptans, and restores an episodic migraine pattern in more than half of the patients. Thus, detoxification is the necessary first step in treatment of rebound.

In most clinical situations, abrupt discontinuation of simple analgesics, triptans, or low amounts of analgesic–caffeine combinations in highly motivated patients without significant psychiatric issues is usually well tolerated. In patients taking barbiturates, opioids, benzodiazepines, or other sedative-containing medications, outpatient detoxification can also be attempted, but under close supervision with a very slow taper.

Inpatient detoxification may be necessary for patients who fail outpatient detoxification or who are consuming large amounts of barbiturates, opioids, or benzodiazepines. These patients may need close supervision or concurrent treatment to prevent withdrawal symptoms. An inpatient setting may also be necessary for a patient who has significant psychological, behavioral, or medical comorbidity.

The patient discussed above had failed prior attempts at detoxification in inpatient settings until a multidisciplinary approach was used to address issues underlying her pattern of drug use. Concomitant behavioral intervention, biofeedback, cognitive behavioral therapy, physical therapy, and nutritional therapy are all part of the multidisciplinary approach needed to relieve the patient's symptoms and prevent a relapse.

Detailed descriptions of detoxification procedures and management of rebound are beyond the scope of this discussion and can be found elsewhere (eg, Raskin, 1986). Long-term prognosis is dependent on many factors and is likely to require comprehensive education regarding the avoidance of behaviors leading to rebound and multidisciplinary supportive follow-up.

Editors' Note

From a historical point of view, credit for the first comprehensive clinical study identifying medication overuse as a causative factor in rebound was the pivotal work by Kudrow at the California Medical Clinic for Headache, published in 1982 and titled *Paradoxical Effects of Analgesic Use*. Most rebound can, in fact, be managed in an outpatient setting by a primary care physician. As Dr. Lucas noted, if multiple medications are being used or there is significant burden of medical and psychiatric comorbid illnesses, referral or inpatient treatment may be necessary.

It is useful to distinguish between addiction (as measured by *Diagnostic and Statistical Manual of Mental Disorders* criteria) and inadvertent habituation associated with anticipatory anxiety, which is experienced by most patients with chronic migraine and medication overuse (the new International Headache Society terminology for rebound). If the primary care physician undertakes detoxification with a rebound patient, only to discover addiction and substance abuse problems, there is not much lost, and appropriate referral can thus be made.

If the patient has straightforward rebound, a gradual taper of rebound medications and a gradual escalation of preventive medications can be started at the same time. Occasionally, we start the preventive medication and gradually build it up to therapeutic levels before beginning detoxification. We provide triptans (if the patient is not in triptan rebound) for rescue use up to 2 days per week during the treatment. We often start daily vitamin B_2 and magnesium, as well as biofeedback or other behavioral therapies. The patient should keep a diary of headaches and medication intake and should be seen frequently.

Diagnosis: Chronic Migraine With Medication Overuse (Rebound Headache)

Selected Reading

Diener HC, Tfelt-Hansen P. Headache associated with chronic use of substances. In: Olesen J, Tfelt-Hansen P, Welch KMA, eds. *The Headaches.* New York, NY: Raven Press; 1993:721-727.

Mathew NT, Kurman R, Perez F. Drug-induced refractory headache—clinical features and management. *Headache.* 1990;30:634-638.

Mathew NT, Reuveni U, Perez F. Transformed or evolutive migraines. *Headache.* 1987;27: 102-106.

Mathew NT, Stubits E, Nigam MP. Transformation of episodic migraine into chronic daily headache: an analysis of factors. *Headache.* 1982;22:66-68.

Rapoport AM. Analgesic rebound headache. *Headache.* 1988;28:662-665.

Raskin NH. Repetitive intravenous dihydroergotamine as therapy for intractable migraine. *Neurology.* 1986;36:995-997.

Saper JR, Jones JM. Ergotamine tartrate dependency. *Clin Neuropharmacol.* 1986;9:244-256.

Silberstein SD, Lipton RB. Chronic daily headache, including transformed migraine, chronic tension-type headache, and medication overuse. In: Silberstein SD, Lipton RB, Dalessio DJ, eds. *Wolff's Headache.* New York, NY: Oxford University Press; 2001:247-282.

Silverman K, Evans SM, Strain EC, et al. Withdrawal syndrome after the double-blind cessation of caffeine consumption. *N Engl J Med.* 1992;327:1109-1114.

Zed PJ, Loewen PS, Robinson G. Medication-induced headache: overview and systematic review of therapeutic approaches. *Ann Pharmacother.* 1999;33:61-72.

7. Patients With Headaches And Neurologic Features

Mark W. Green, MD

Clinical Professor of Neurology
Columbia University College of Physicians and Surgeons
New York, New York

Case 1

A 38-year-old woman was referred by her internist for complaints of "numbness."

She had a long-established, stereotypical history of strange feelings, on one side of her body, that occurred every few weeks. She described a tingling of the left hand extending up her left arm over a period of approximately 20 minutes. As it moved toward the face, the hand felt numb. A tingling feeling occurred on the left side of the mouth and tongue, replaced in minutes by a numb feeling. Often this would be followed by a mild throbbing headache on the left side, accompanied by nausea and photophobia, lasting about 4 to 6 hours.

Past Medical History

Unremarkable.

Family History

Significant for headache in several members who had never been diagnosed.

Neurologic Exam

Normal.

Case 2

A 72-year-old man with no previous history of headache presented with 3 episodes of numbness that had occurred over the previous 2 weeks. He described an abrupt onset of numbness of the left side of his face, with progression to the entire left arm within approximately 1 minute. His family noted some clumsiness and weakness of his left arm and leg during the attack. A pounding headache on the right side accompanied the numbness at onset. All symptoms resolved in approximately 4 hours.

Past Medical History

Significant for hypercholesterolemia and hypertension. The man had been relatively noncompliant with medications, which included a statin and a diuretic.

Family History

Negative for headache, but positive for premature coronary artery disease in his father and paternal uncle.

Exam

His neurologic exam showed a subtle left-sided drift with some intention tremor.

Discussion

Migraine with aura occurs in 15% to 30% of migraineurs, and is often a dramatic and frightening event. Visual disturbances occur in 90% of all migraineurs with aura. The onset of aura is often peripubertal. Unlike the old terminology of "classic migraine," which referred only to visual auras, the International Headache Society (IHS) classification of "migraine with aura" includes all of the focal neurologic complaints accompanying the headache of migraine as "aura" (Table, page 60).

Aura tends to precede but may accompany the attack of head pain. Most auras develop over a few minutes and last 20 to 30 minutes, although the IHS criteria allow for a duration of typical aura symptoms of up to 1 hour.

Initially, visual auras tend to involve a small portion of the visual field and then extend, increasing in size and moving across the visual field. Since all focal symptomatology associated with a migraine attack is considered to be an aura, the IHS classification does not distinguish between visual aura, hemisensory abnormality, ataxia, hemiparesis, and disturbances of consciousness, awareness, or language.

Visual disturbances, the most common form of migraine aura, vary widely and include multicolored dots in both visual fields, photopsias (light flashes, or "phosphenes"), fortification spectra (teichopsia or zigzags), various scotomata or blind spots, mosaic vision (like looking through a kaleidoscope), and metamorphotic changes such as micropsia (small distortions) and macropsia (large distortions).

Migraine headache pain, when present, follows the aura within 1 hour (typically within 5 to 15 minutes).

Although a variety of focal complaints can occur with headache and may be caused by migraine, other, more serious neurologic conditions can mimic the migraine aura. Among patients with transient ischemic attacks or stroke, 30% will experience headache, most commonly when the event involves the vertebrobasilar distribution. It is often problematic, although important, to differentiate these more serious conditions, which have very different degrees of significance for the patient. This is particularly true for the 72-year-old man in Case 2.

Differentiating aura from other neurologic conditions requires an understanding of migraine pathophysiology. Many physicians were taught the Wolff Vascular Theory of Migraine, which attributed aura to vasoconstriction of intracranial arteries, which in turn produced ischemic symptoms. The headache was then thought to be due to a rebound vasodilation of superficial temporal vessels, with subsequent recovery in blood flow.

However, we know that headaches can begin simultaneously with aura, making it unlikely that symptoms are explained by alterations in blood vessel caliber. This theory never addressed many of the phases of migraine that suggest the cortex and the brain stem are involved in the generation of a migraine attack.

The slow progression of migrainous visual auras was described in detail by Airy in 1870 and by Gowers in 1906. Lashley, a neurologist suffering from migraine, observed in 1941 the detailed movement of his own migrainous fortification spectrum across the visual field. He calculated that this cortical event spread across his cerebral cortex at the rate of 3 mm per minute and was followed by a wave of total inhibition. Lashley noted that the scotoma was exceedingly bright, comparing it to a white surface reflecting the sun at noon. Leão, a neurophysiologist working at Harvard in 1944, found that a variety of techniques that stimulated the exposed cerebral cortex of animals caused a positive wave to propagate across the cortex (at 2 to 3 mm per minute). He observed that this positive wave, reflecting hyperexcitability of the cortex, left behind a prolonged wave of inhibition. This has been referred to as cortical spreading depression (CSD).

The aura symptoms themselves are probably due to excitation of neurons. Following the excitation, the cortical neurons become relatively silent, and require less blood flow, resulting in a wave of oligemia spreading anteriorly at the same rate as the CSD found in animals. Oligemia is not ischemia, and this period is likely asymptomatic.

It should not be assumed that migraines with and without aura can be distinguished by means of these physiologic changes. It is possible that many more migraines are associated with aura than are recognized, yet the brain regions involved are silent or cause only vague symptoms. Woods et al were able to measure the regional blood flow of a 21-year-old woman who had clinical migraine without aura. In a spontaneous attack while in a positron emission tomography scanner, the woman developed bilateral reduction in cerebral blood flow starting in the occiput and moving anteriorly unaccompanied by any symptoms. Two other authors have reported similar cases.

Nonetheless, some believe that migraine with and without aura are separate disorders with different underlying genetic determinants. Russell et al recently performed a population-based twin survey and determined that

Table. The International Headache Society Criteria for Migraine With Aura

A. At least 2 attacks fulfilling (B)

B. At least 3 of the following 4 characteristics:

- One or more fully reversible aura symptoms indicating brain dysfunction;
- At least 1 aura symptom develops gradually over more than 4 minutes, or 2 or more symptoms occur in succession;
- No single aura symptom lasts more than 60 minutes;
- Headache follows aura with a free interval of less than 60 minutes (or simultaneously with the aura).

C. History, physical examination, and—where appropriate—diagnostic tests exclude a secondary cause concurrence of migraine with and without aura in twins was the same as the prevalence in the general population. This suggests that these are distinct disorders. It is certain, however, that migraine with and without aura is multifactorial in origin and that multiple genes and multiple environmental triggers interact to produce an attack of migraine. If these 2 conditions are genetically distinct, it is difficult to explain why those experiencing migraine with aura often have similar attacks without aura.

It is best to understand a migraineur as having a "hypersensitive brain" in much the same way that individuals with asthma have hypersensitive bronchial airways. Most migraineurs will report a lifelong sensitivity to stress, lights, smells, sounds, and various foods, as well as impaired sleep. Migraineurs will be unusually sensitive to various visual stimuli, which can include striped patterns on clothes or fluorescent lighting. This hypersensitivity can also be demonstrated by transcranial magnetic stimulation. If such a stimulator is applied to the scalp over the occipital cortex and a sufficient degree of stimulation is applied, all subjects, whether or not they have a history of migraine, will see phosphenes. Those with migraine will visualize phosphenes with far less magnetic stimulation than those without migraine.

Aura Versus TIA and Secondary Causes

Distinguishing a migraine aura with headache from a transient ischemic attack or cerebral infarction with headache may be possible on clinical grounds. A migrainous aura will commonly cause a positive symptom to "travel," leaving behind in its trail a negative symptom. An example would be a small scintillation in a visual field, which, as it expands, leaves behind a blind spot. Tingling that progresses down the face and then the arm, resolving but leaving behind an underlying numb sensation, would be analogous.

Sensory auras are the most common auras after visual auras. Characteristically, they are cheiro-oral. This means that the numbness usually begins in the hand, marches up the arm, and then involves the lips, mouth, and tongue. As would be predictable from the physiology of spreading depression, there are often positive phenomena. For example, as paresthesias spread, they lead to negative phenomena such as numbness. The woman in Case 1 exhibited a march of symptoms typical of migraine, with a duration typical of migraine. The fact that her headache was ipsilateral to her symptoms may also be more consistent with migraine than a cerebral ischemic event.

What comprises an appropriate evaluation of a migraine aura is, at times, difficult to determine. The reason for this is the way that headaches change with the addition of secondary syndromes. When a long-term headache sufferer develops a secondary cause of headache—for example, a brain tumor—it may retain the pattern of the original headache type. If a patient with a known history of migraine with aura develops a tumor, it can manifest by an increase in migraines with aura, rather than the development of a new headache. A substantial increase in the frequency of migraine attacks or their intensity over time should prompt a re-evaluation. A change in the pattern of headache, with or without an increase in frequency or intensity, is a cause for concern, and further workup should be considered, depending on clinical presentation.

The man in Case 2 had spells that were likely due to transient ischemic attacks (TIAs), not migraine with aura. The march of symptoms was very brief, and the attacks of short duration. TIA symptoms tend to have a more apoplectic onset than those of migraine. Focal symptoms in a TIA tend to occur over approximately 1 minute and have a usual duration of less than 15 minutes. The cheiro-oral march characteristic of migraine is unusual in TIA.

Motor symptoms, such as hemipareses, occur rarely in migraine and are generally unilateral. More commonly in migraine patients, weakness is a misperception of numbness; when tested, the patient has normal strength. Transient focal neurologic symptoms can be seen in association with, or dissociated from, migraine headaches (see Aurora chapter, page 105). Neurologic symptoms as part of aura can be diagnosed with more confidence when they also occur in association with headache.

Migraine is a risk factor for the development of ischemic stroke, but migraine with aura appears to confer a higher risk, with an odds ratio of 2:1 to 3:1 in women younger than age 40. Doubling or tripling the very low stroke risk in this population, however, still results in a very tiny risk.

However, cigarette smoking and the use of oral contraceptives further increase this risk. For this reason, estrogen-containing oral contraceptives are contraindicated in women who smoke cigarettes and experience migraine with aura. Women with any type of migraine should be warned about smoking and should be given the facts about the role of estrogen.

From 20% to 60% of migraine attacks are preceded by a prodrome, which can begin up to 1 day before other migraine symptoms. The prodrome often consists of vague symptoms of fatigue, mood changes, frequent urination, hunger, or yawning. Prodromes are not part of the IHS criteria for diagnosing migraine or aura, and need to be distinguished from aura.

There is some evidence that the migraine prodromes may involve dopaminergic pathways, originating in the hypothalamus. If a dopamine antagonist is administered during a prodrome, the entire attack can be prevented.

Serotonin may also be involved. Cady et al demonstrated that naratriptan (Amerge), administered during a migraine prodrome, can prevent a migraine attack.

As noted in the discussion of Case 2, migraine is not the cause of all focal neurologic events associated with headache. Along with TIAs, carotid or vertebral dissections, arteriovenous malformations, neoplasms, and even partial seizures should be considered. It has been stated for many years that if the aura is stereotyped and lateralized to a fixed location, a secondary headache should be a serious consideration. Certainly cases of occipital arteriovenous malformations with a stereotyped and lateralized aura have been seen. In other cases, arteriovenous malformations have been associated with auras that change sides with various attacks.

Thus, structural disorders that mimic migraine, such as neoplasms and arteriovenous malformations, may simply be other triggers of migraine in a genetically predisposed individual. I have seen several migraineurs experiencing aura associated with arteriovenous malformations who have no change in their migraine attacks after treatment of the malformation.

Migraine is not the only primary headache that has been associated with aura. Although rare, cases of cluster headache and hemicrania continua associated with typical visual auras have also been reported.

Treatment

Treatment of aura is difficult. Antimigraine agents have been developed to treat the migraine headache pain. Many also treat the associated nausea, vomiting, photophobia, and phonophobia, but none has been shown to abort the aura. The Wolff theory raised concern that all vasoactive antimigraine drugs, such as ergots and triptans, might extend or prolong an aura. This has not been found in prospective studies. Triptans and ergots apparently neither worsen nor relieve the aura, which means they are probably safe to use in the presence of a typical aura. However, triptans have not demonstrated efficacy in aborting aura or treating the migraine headache that follows, although most studies have been small and possibly underpowered. Most specialists recommend having patients wait until their aura is over before treating with a triptan. When injectable sumatriptan (Imitrex) was administered during aura to document safety, the aura was unchanged and the headache was not prevented. In cases in which the headache historically does not follow the aura, it is best to wait and see if the headache actually develops before treatment is initiated. Other specialists believe that in cases where the aura always precedes the headache and the headache occurs at least 30 minutes after the start of the aura, it should be possible to use oral triptans early in the aura to prevent or reduce the headache that follows.

Hemiplegic migraine and basilar migraine are contraindications to use of triptans and ergots, as migraineurs with these syndromes were excluded in the clinical trials. However, until further proof is forthcoming about the safety of triptans in these conditions, they should remain contraindicated. Isolated "dizziness" is widely seen in migraine attacks and does not constitute a diagnosis of basilar migraine (see Levin chapter, page 65).

Sensory auras were seen in many patients during triptan clinical trials and are well studied. They should not preclude therapy with triptans. There is no evidence that any acutely administered migraine therapy worsens migraine auras.

Low brain magnesium levels have been documented by nuclear magnetic resonance spectroscopy and may play a role in the cortical hypersensitivity seen in migraine. Supplementing the diet with magnesium may be of value in some patients. Otherwise, the treatment of migraine with aura is the same as the treatment of migraine without aura. More treatments of aura are described in the chapter by Dr. Aurora.

Editors' Note

Stereotypical neurologic symptoms lasting less than 1 hour, followed within 1 hour by headache, constitute criteria for migraine with aura. Dr. Green provides 2 cases as bookends. One is that of an established pattern in a menstruating woman of benign sensory symptoms of 20-minute durations, followed invariably by classic migraine with aura.

But in an elderly man whose symptoms are abrupt in onset and persistent for 4 hours, benign migraine with aura is unlikely, and TIA should be considered. Further clues include an absence of family history, absence of personal history of migraine until age 72, vascular risk factors, and abnormal findings on focal exam. The change in pattern, sudden onset, long duration, and gender and age of the patient all suggest a different diagnosis.

Dr. Green also describes optimal use of triptans in migraine with aura: after the aura and at the beginning of pain. In the man with TIAs, the pain and neurologic features occurred simultaneously, which is unusual in aura and might give a clinician a clue to the necessity of workup.

<u>Diagnoses:</u> Case 1, Migraine With Aura; Case 2, Transient Ischemic Attack

Selected Reading

Airy H. On a distinct form of transient hemianopsia. *Philosophical Transactions of the Royal Society of London*. 1870;160:247-264.

Aurora SK, Cao Y, Bowyer SM, Welch KMA. The occipital cortex is hyperexcitable in migraine: experimental. *Headache*. 1999;39:469-476.

Bank J. Migraine with aura after administration of sublingual nitroglycerine. *Headache*. 2001;41:84-87.

Bates D, Ashford E, Dawson R, et al. Subcutaneous sumatriptan during the migraine aura. *Neurology*. 1994;44:1587-1592.

De Benedittis G, Ferrari Da Passano C, Granata G, Lorenzitti A. CBF changes during headache-free periods and spontaneous/induced attacks in migraine with and without aura: a TCD and SPECT comparison study. *J Neurosurg Sci*. 1999;43:141-146.

Fisher CM. Late-life accompaniments as a cause of unexplained transient ischemic attacks. Dutch RIA Study Group. *Stroke*. 1991;22:754-759.

Gelmers HJ. Common migraine attacks preceded by focal hyperemia and parietal oligemia in the rCBF pattern. *Cephalalgia*. 1982;2:29-32.

Gowers WR. Clinical lectures on the borderland of epilepsy. *Br Med J*. 1906;2:1617-1622.

Lauritzen M, Skyhoj-Olsen T, Lassen NA, Pauson OB. Regulation of regional cerebral blood flow during and between migraine attacks. *Ann Neurol*. 1983;14:569-572.

Leão AAP. Spreading depression of activity in cerebral cortex. *J Neurophysiol*. 1944;7:358-390.

Mulleners WM, Chronicle EP, Palmer JE, et al. Visual cortex excitability in migraine with and without aura. *Headache*. 2001;41:565-572.

Olesen J, Friberg L, Skyhoj-Olsen T, et al. Timing and topography of cerebral blood flow, aura and headache during migraine attacks. *Ann Neurol*. 1990;28:791-798.

Russell MB, Ulrich V, Gervil M, Olesen J. Migraine without aura and migraine with aura are distinct disorders: a population-based twin survey. *Headache*. 2002;42:332-336.

Welch KMA, D'Andrea G, Tepley N, Barkeley GL, Ramadan NM. The concept of migraine as a state of central neuronal hyperexcitability. *Headache*. 1990;8:817-828.

Wijman CA, Wolf PA, Kase CS, at al. Migrainous visual accompaniments are not rare in late life: the Framingham Study. *Stroke*. 1998;29:1539-1543.

Woods RP, Iacoboni M, Mazziotta JC. Bilateral spreading cerebral hypoperfusion during spontaneous migraine headache. *N Engl J Med*. 1994;331:1689-1692.

8. The Patient With Headache And Dizziness

Morris Levin, MD

Assistant Professor
Departments of Medicine (Neurology) and Psychiatry
Dartmouth Medical School
Co-director, Dartmouth Headache Center
Dartmouth-Hitchcock Medical Center
Lebanon, New Hampshire

Case

A 51-year-old woman was referred by her primary care physician with the complaint of dizziness.

Her doctor had diagnosed vertigo. Intermittent vertigo, described as a sensation of movement of herself or her surroundings, had been bothering her for several years. Over the previous 3 to 4 months, the sensation had worsened in severity and duration until it was nearly constant.

Her symptoms were often accompanied by nausea, "dimming of vision," lightheadedness, and an unpleasant feeling of head "fullness." Head position changes worsened symptoms only slightly. Vomiting occurred rarely, but her nausea was often disabling.

The vertigo and head fullness failed to respond to a number of medications, including meclizine, antihistamines, antiemetics, amitriptyline, and valproate (Depakote). Some of her medication trials were terminated within days to weeks because of either adverse effects or lack of effectiveness.

Since early childhood, the patient had experienced unilateral throbbing headaches accompanied by nausea, blurring of vision, and vertigo. The headaches began to occur approximately once every 2 months and lasted around 2 days. Oral sumatriptan (Imitrex) 50 mg was quite effective in aborting her headaches, and she felt that the low headache frequency was due to her current preventive program of atenolol 25 mg daily and alprazolam 0.5 mg twice daily.

Past Medical History

Remarkable for hyperthyroidism and gastritis. She had been pregnant twice and delivered 2 children without complications.

Review of Systems

Remarkable for chronic intermittent neck pain and poor sleep marked by frequent awakening. She had seen a number of specialists for evaluation of dizziness, headache, and neck pain, and had been diagnosed with fibromyalgia, temporomandibular joint dysfunction, benign positional vertigo, migraine, and tension headaches. Her menstrual periods are irregular, and have been so for a number of years.

Diagnostic Evaluation

Included a brain magnetic resonance image (MRI) that revealed one small area of signal change in the right centrum semiovale, and a cervical MRI showing a bulging C6-C7 disk without spinal cord or foraminal encroachment.

Family History

Remarkable for headaches in the patient's 2 children (30 and 32 years old). Neither complained of vertigo, and there was no other family history of headache, vertigo, or neurologic problems.

Social History and Habits

The patient is married, works as a medical billing specialist, and exercises sporadically. She does not smoke or drink alcohol. She drinks 1 cup of coffee daily.

Current Medications

Alprazolam 0.5 mg bid; atenolol 25 mg daily; thyroid replacement; pravastatin (Pravachol).

General Medical Examination

A physical examination revealed the subject to be a healthy woman with a blood pressure reading of 120/82 and regular pulse of 64. Neck was supple, and carotid auscultation was normal. Posterior cervical muscle tightness was noted, with some tenderness in splenius capitus and occipitalis regions. Ophthalmoscopic findings were normal. Lungs were clear, and cardiac and abdominal examinations yielded normal results. Skin was normal.

Neurologic Exam

Normal findings, including mental status, cranial nerves, motor tone and strength, reflexes, sensation, coordination, and gait. Specifically, facial nerve function was normal, hearing was excellent, and nystagmus was absent. Hallpike maneuver failed to worsen vertigo or induce nystagmus, but the subject did become slightly dysphoric with head position below horizontal.

Discussion

A relationship between migraine and vertigo has been noted and discussed for many years. Most headache specialists have noted a common type of labyrinthine/vestibular symptom in a subset of their migraine patients, from a mild feeling of dysequilibrium or particular sensitivity to motion, to profound disabling vertigo in conjunction with headache. However, since migraine is common (affecting some 12% of the population) and dizziness even more so (about 20% in the general population), the statistical validity of an association has been questioned.

There is also the problem of many different definitions and perceptions of vertigo and dizziness among patients and practitioners (Table 1). Even so, vertigo has been found to be approximately 3 times as common in migraine patients as in the general population, and migraine has been found to be significantly more common in patients seen for complaints of vertigo. Lesion localization targets for vertigo are listed in Table 2.

Table 1. Symptoms Associated With Dizziness

- Anxiety
- Blurred vision
- Disorientation
- Imbalance
- Light-headedness (presyncope)
- Vertigo

The International Headache Society (IHS) classification of migraine includes vertigo as a symptom only in the basilar migraine category, and does not specify a category of migrainous vertigo. Migraine-associated vertigo continues to be diagnosed frequently, though, in dizziness clinics and otolaryngologists' offices around the world, when other causes of recurrent vestibular symptoms have all been excluded.

In a prospective study of the interrelation between migraine and vertigo, Neuhauser and his team at the Neurologische Klinik of Humboldt-Universität in Berlin found that migraine was significantly more common in patients seen in their dizziness clinic than in controls. They defined a category termed "migrainous vertigo" as including 1) episodic vestibular symptoms of at least moderate severity, 2) migraine according to IHS criteria, 3) some migrainous symptoms during at least some of the vertiginous attacks, and 4) no other cause of vestibulopathy. They identified several patients with this condition; of interest, none fulfilled the IHS criteria for migraine with aura.

In patients seeking medical advice for recurrent vertigo with or without headaches, a number of diagnostic entities must be excluded (Table 3, page 68). Most important, masses in the region of the cerebellopontine angle and inflammatory or infectious processes in the subarachnoid space must not be missed, but are usually excluded by exam and imaging procedures.

When hearing loss accompanies recurrent bouts of vertigo, Meniere's disease becomes more likely, and here headache can be a concomitant symptom. Benign positional vertigo and posttraumatic vertigo can both occur in combination with recurrent headaches.

In the patient described above, the diagnosis of migraine-associated vertigo is apt. Episodic vestibular symptoms were the primary complaint. Some episodes, but certainly not all, were associated with migraine head pain. IHS criteria for migraine were met. Examination did not suggest any other neurologic disease, and provocative testing for vestibular pathology proved negative. Neuroimaging failed to identify a labyrinthine or vestibular system site of pathology.

Table 2. Lesion Localization in Vertigo

- Cerebellum
- Cortical centers
- Labyrinths
- Vestibular nuclei in brain stem
- VIII nerve

Table 3. Differential Diagnosis of Vertigo

1. Benign positional vertigo
2. Medication effect (aspirin, phenytoin, aminoglycosides, cisplatin)
3. Vestibular neuronitis (labyrinthitis)
4. Meniere's disease
5. Posttraumatic vertigo
6. Phobic vertigo
7. Perilymphatic fistula
8. Neurosyphilis
9. Meningitis (carcinomatous, tuberculosis, fungal, bacterial)
10. Sarcoidosis
11. CNS vasculitis
12. Ramsay Hunt syndrome (zoster infection of geniculate ganglion)
13. Cogan's syndrome (keratitis, vertigo, ataxia, nystagmus, hearing loss)
14. Intralabyrinthine hemorrhage (leukemia, trauma)
15. Acoustic neuroma and other cerebellopontile angle tumors, meningioma, epidermoid, cholesteatoma, metastatic tumor
16. Compression of the acoustic nerve by ectatic artery (microvascular compression)
17. Multiple sclerosis (brain-stem plaque)
18. Brain-stem neoplasm or arteriovenous malformations
19. Brain-stem ischemia
20. Complex partial seizure ("tornado seizure")
21. Migrainous vertigo

Treatment

In a very detailed and complete review, Glenn Johnson, at Dartmouth-Hitchcock Medical Center in Lebanon, NH, proposed a multifactorial approach to the treatment of migraine-related vertigo, including all typical migraine prophylactic agents, benzodiazepines (which exert their effects on gamma-aminobutyric acid systems found throughout the vestibular system), and selective serotonin reuptake inhibitor medications such as sertraline (Zoloft). He also stressed the importance of nonpharmacologic treatments such as dietary changes, physical therapy, and lifestyle adaptation.

In his 1998 article, Dr. Johnson described a retrospective review of patients diagnosed with "migraine-related dizziness and vertigo." Using the approaches described, he achieved complete or substantial control of vestibular symptoms in approximately 90% of patients.

In the patient described above, a repeat MRI scan with gadolinium failed to reveal any pathology in the cerebellopontile angle, audiologic evaluation remained entirely normal, and neurologic review of systems and examination continued to be unremarkable. She was started on nortriptyline 25 mg qhs, which was later increased to 50 mg qhs. This resulted in significant reduction in vertiginous symptoms as well as reduction in headache frequency and severity. Clonazepam 0.5 mg on a prn basis, used sparingly, is effective for episodic vertigo. Recommendations were made to further evaluate the sleep dysfunction, and for physical therapy aimed at addressing the cervical muscle spasm and local pain.

The relationship between migraine and vertigo can be an especially important one, for several reasons. First, if a patient's vertigo is due to a migrainous etiology, treatment options not generally employed by otologists may be dramatically effective. Second, study of this subset of migraine patients may shed some light on migraine and migraine aura pathophysiology. And, most important for the group of patients who have been misdiagnosed as having "functional" or "psychogenic" vertigo, assigning the correct diagnosis can be an enormous relief.

Editors' Note

The vertigo in migrainous vertigo is probably a manifestation of aura, a neurologic dysfunction lasting less than 1 hour and followed within 60 minutes by headache or head "discomfort." Migraine-specific therapy is standard for both abortive and preventive treatment. This would mean triptans as acute care medications, and tricyclics, ß-blockers, and antiepileptic drugs for prevention. Robert Baloh, MD, a vertigo and dizziness specialist in Los Angeles, has stated that many patients with Meniere's disease, who have vertigo and loss of hearing, actually have migraine.

Diagnosis: Migraine-Associated Vertigo

Selected Reading

Headache Classification Committee of the International Headache Society. Classification & Diagnostic Criteria for Headache Disorders, Cranial Neuralgias and Facial Pain. *Cephalalgia.* 1988;8(suppl 7):1-96.

Johnson GD. Medical management of migraine-related dizziness and vertigo. *Laryngoscope.* 1998;108(1, part 2):1-28.

Neuhauser H Leopold M, von Brevern M, Arnold G, Lempert T. The interrelations of migraine, vertigo, and migrainous vertigo. *Neurology.* 2001;56:436-441.

9. The Woman With Headaches During Her Period

Lawrence C. Newman, MD

Director, the Headache Institute at
St. Luke's–Roosevelt Hospital Center,
New York, New York
Associate Clinical Professor of Neurology
Albert Einstein College of Medicine
Bronx, New York

Case

The patient, a 32-year-old woman, was referred for headaches that had begun in her teens.

Her headaches were described as a throbbing or pressure sensation that began behind one eye and then rapidly spread to the ipsilateral temple. Although the headaches usually occurred on the left side, on rare occasions they were right-sided. The severity of pain ranged from moderate to severe, and the pain often began within 1 hour of waking. The headaches were associated with photophobia and phonophobia and tended to worsen with movement.

During her teens, the patient's headaches had always been associated with nausea and vomiting. For the past 10 years, although nauseated, she no longer vomited with her headaches. She felt an overwhelming sense of exhaustion and craved sweets the night before most of her headaches.

When she was younger, the subject had missed an average of 1 day of school per month because of her headaches, having to remain in her bedroom with the lights out and the shades drawn. Her pediatrician recommended treating the pain with ice packs and acetaminophen, which afforded little or no relief. She believed the headaches resolved on their own, usually within 12 hours of onset.

Her headaches were often triggered by stress, weather changes, and too little sleep, but these triggers were not consistent. Each month, however, usually 1 to 2 days before the onset of menstruation, the patient experienced a severe headache that could last for up to 2 days. These headaches were more severe than her other headaches and occurred each month.

Over the years, the subject's headaches have recurred at varying intervals. During her 2 pregnancies, however, she was relatively headache-free.

At the present time, she reports 2 or 3 headaches monthly, one always in association with her menses. Because of these headaches, she consulted with her gynecologist, who recommended treatment of the acute attacks with naproxen sodium. However, the treatment worsened the nausea. He then gave the subject a prescription for a combination product containing acetaminophen, butalbital, and caffeine, which made her drowsy but did not abort the headaches.

Past Medical History

Unremarkable.

Family History
Positive for a mother and grandmother with "sick" headaches.

Medical and Neurologic Examinations
Normal.

Diagnostic Workup
The subject has never undergone a neuroimaging procedure.

Discussion
Attacks of migraine headache can occur before, during, or after the onset of menstruation. Many women list menstruation as a potent trigger of their migraines. In general, migraine attacks during menstruation tend not to be associated with aura, are of a longer duration, are more resistant to therapy, and tend to recur after treatment.

Currently, there is no universally accepted definition of menstrual migraine (MM). In general, MM encompasses 2 subtypes: "true" menstrual migraine and "menstrually associated" migraine.

"True" menstrual migraine implies that migraine attacks occur exclusively during the menstrual period and at no other time during the month. "True" MM is rare, affecting 7% to 14% of women migraineurs.

"Menstrually associated" migraine (MAM) is defined as migraine attacks that are not limited to the menses; these patients report headaches at other times during the month in addition to attacks during menstruation. This migraine subtype is reported by approximately 60% to 70% of women migraineurs. It is generally accepted that MAM usually occurs from day –2 to day +3, where onset of menses is designated day 0.

MMs occur at the time of the largest fluctuations of estrogen levels. Somerville found that MMs occurred either during or after the decline in levels of both estrogens and progesterone. Because premenstrual administration of estrogen will delay the headache but not the timing of the menstruation, whereas progesterone administration delays menstruation without preventing migraine, it is presumed that it is the withdrawal of estrogen that triggers the migraine.

The current patient's headaches meet the International Headache Society criteria for migraine without aura. As her headaches occur in association with her menses, as well as other times of the month, she can be given the diagnosis of MAM, although this subclassification of migraine is not recognized in the International Headache Society (IHS) classification.

Treatment
The management of MM is in large part similar to the treatment of migraine in general. Medications that are efficacious in the acute treatment of migraine are also useful in the treatment of MM. These include the nonsteroidal anti-inflammatory drugs (NSAIDs) such as ibuprofen, naproxen sodium, meclofenamate, and indomethacin; dihydroergotamine, a nonselective 5-HT$_1$ agonist that can be given parenterally (D.H.E. 45) or as a nasal spray (Migranal); oral ergotamine tartrate preparations (Cafergot); and com-

binations of aspirin, acetaminophen, and caffeine (Excedrin). The selective 5-HT$_{1B/D}$ agonists, the triptans, are as effective for MAM as for nonmenstrually associated migraine. Sumatriptan (Imitrex), zolmitriptan (Zomig), and rizatriptan (Maxalt) are especially useful for MAM associated with nausea and vomiting.

Women suffering from frequent, disabling migraine attacks may also be candidates for preventive therapy. For women prescribed preventive medications for migraine who continue to suffer from MAM, transiently increasing the dose of their daily medications immediately before their menses can sometimes prevent or lessen the severity of MAM.

For women with "true" menstrual migraine and those whose migraines associated with their menses occur at regular intervals, a short-term preventive strategy may be employed. The best way to determine if in fact migraines are related to menstruation is to have patients fill out diaries in which they log when headaches and menstruation occur. In this way, the physician can accurately estimate the timing of these headaches and plan a prophylactic strategy.

For women who have regular menstrual cycles and whose diaries demonstrate a predictable pattern of MAM, several perimenstrual dosing strategies are possible. Medications that employ a short-term prophylactic regimen include NSAIDs, ergotamine tartrate, dihydroergotamine, the triptans, and magnesium. Naproxen sodium 550 mg bid beginning 1 to 2 days before the anticipated onset of the headache and continued throughout the duration of the menses is a well-described treatment strategy.

The efficacy of ergotamine tartrate bid or dihydroergotamine nasal spray every 8 hours, beginning 3 days before the expected onset of migraine and continued for a total of 6 days, has also been reported. Perimenstrual supplementation of magnesium was found to decrease the duration and severity of MM.

In an open-label trial of sumatriptan 25 mg tid beginning 2 to 3 days before the expected onset of headache and continued for 5 days, headache was absent in 52% of subjects; 42% reported a 50% or greater reduction in headache severity. A recent double-blind, placebo-controlled trial of naratriptan reported that 1 mg bid 2 days before expected headache onset and continued for 5 days was statistically superior to placebo in reducing the number of MAM headache days and headache severity.

For MAM unresponsive to the above-mentioned therapies, hormonal treatments may be necessary. The perimenstrual application of an estrogen patch (0.5 or 1.0 mg applied 1 to 2 days before the onset of headache and continued for 5 days) has been reported to prevent MM, as has continuous oral contraceptive use without interruption for up to 4 months at a time.

There is no evidence that treatments with diuretics or surgical treatments such as hysterectomy or oophorectomy are of any value in the management of MM.

As our patient has a long-standing history of migraine that meets IHS criteria for migraine without aura, and has headaches that alternate sides between attacks, a strong family history of migraine, and normal results of medical and neurologic examinations, there is no need to order a neuroimaging procedure. Additionally, there is no information to gain in obtaining serum estrogen levels in a young, otherwise healthy woman, since no evidence exists that MAM results from abnormal hormone levels.

Management Strategies
- Have the patient track headache and menstrual cycles by keeping a headache diary. This will verify whether a menstrual association is present and document when during the cycle headaches occur. Diaries can also identify other potential migraine triggers.
- Determine whether the headaches are strictly limited to the menstrual cycle or, as is more common, occur with the menses and at other times.
- Treat individual attacks with standard antimigraine medications (NSAIDs, ergots, triptans, etc).
- For medically resistant cases of MM, consider short-term preventive strategies with NSAIDs, ergots, or triptans.
- If headache frequency is high (more than 6 days monthly), preventive medications may be warranted.
- Hormonal manipulation should be reserved for the most treatment-refractory patients.
- Diuretics, hysterectomy, and oophorectomy have no role in the treatment of MM.

Editors' Note
Dr. Newman provides a commonsense approach to managing menstrual migraine. The first issue confronted is diagnosis, which he favors cementing with use of a headache diary. We favor the –2- to +3-day definition of menstrually associated migraine; if a patient's migraines are not in the window and are not locked to flow, miniprevention strategies are not practical. Then he lists the strategies themselves; we favor the order of an NSAID trial, followed by a triptan trial, with hormonal manipulation as the last resort.

<u>Diagnosis:</u> Menstrually Associated Migraine

Selected Reading
Bousser MG, Massiou H. Migraine in the reproductive cycle. In: Olesen J, Tfelt-Hansen P, Welch KMA, eds. *The Headaches*. New York, NY: Raven Press;1993:413-420.

Diamond S, Freitag FG, Diamond ML, et al. Subcutaneous dihydroergotamine mesylate (DHE) in the treatment of menstrual migraine. *Headache Q.* 1996;7:145-147.

Lay CL, Newman LC. Menstrual migraine: approaches to management. *CNS Drugs.* 1999; 12:189-195.

Loder E, Silberstein S. Clinical efficacy of 2.5 and 5 mg zolmitriptan in migraine associated with menses or in patients using non-progestogen oral contraceptives. *Neurology.* 1998; 50(Suppl 4):A341.

Loder E, Silberstein S, Giammarco R, et al. Oral zolmitriptan exhibits efficacy as early as 30 minutes in menstrually associated migraine: results of a large multicenter placebo-controlled study. *Neurology.* 2002;58(Suppl 3):A414-A415.

Newman L, Mannix LK, Landy S, et al. Naratriptan as short-term prophylaxis of menstrually associated migraine: a randomized, double-blind, placebo-controlled study. *Headache.* 2000;41:248-256.

Newman LC, Lipton RB, Lay CL, Solomon S. A pilot study of oral sumatriptan as intermittent prophylaxis of menstruation-related migraine. *Neurology*. 1998;51:307-309.

Salonen R, Saiers J. Sumatriptan is effective in the treatment of menstrual migraine: a review of prospective studies and retrospective analyses. *Cephalalgia*. 1999;19:16-19.

Sances G, Martigononi E, Fioroni L, et al. Naproxen sodium in menstrual migraine prophylaxis: a double blind placebo controlled study. *Headache*. 1990;30:705-709.

Silberstein SD. D.H.E. 45 in the prophylaxis of menstrually related migraine. *Cephalalgia*. 1996;16:371.

Silberstein SD. Menstrual migraine. *J Womens Health Gend Based Med*. 1999;8:919-931.

Silberstein SD, Massiou H, LeJunne C, et al. Rizatriptan in the treatment of menstrual migraine. *Obstet Gynecol*. 2000;96:237-242.

Silberstein SD, Merriam GR. Sex hormones and headache. *J Pain Symptom Manage*. 1993;8:98-114.

Somerville BW. Estrogen-withdrawal migraine: attempted prophylaxis by continuous estradiol administration. *Neurology*. 1975;25:245-250.

10. The Woman With Left TMJ Pain

Steven Graff-Radford, DDS

Co-director, The Pain Center
Cedars-Sinai Medical Center
San Vicente, California

Case

A 42-year-old woman presented with intermittent pain in the left preauricular area radiating to the temple. The pain was described as sharp and achy and sometimes pulsing. It occurred randomly, as often as twice a week.

The pain could last many hours and, when severe, could be associated with nausea and photophobia. The subject complained of noise in the left temporomandibular joint when she opened her mouth wide, and felt this worsened with extensive chewing.

The patient reported she had been experiencing these symptoms intermittently since she was in college. She reported worsening during stressful situations and during menses. She obtained relief by placing cold compresses over the face and temple.

The subject had sought evaluations from her dentist, who diagnosed a temporomandibular disorder (TMD) and treated her with an intraoral bite splint. She thought it helped initially, but then it seemed the pain occurred despite appropriate use of the splint.

Her primary care doctor felt that the pain was stress related and prescribed alprazolam, to be used as needed. The patient found this helped her to sleep, but did not stop the pain.

She was then referred to an ear, nose, and throat specialist and for some time seemed to obtain relief from a combination of analgesics and decongestants. A holistic approach was also attempted, without benefit.

Past Medical History and Review of Systems

Normal except for the report of some difficulty falling asleep, which she attributed to the pain. She was not depressed or anxious.

Medication History

The subject was not taking any medication except for pain relievers. She reported using an over-the-counter anti-inflammatory medication once or twice a week. This did not provide significant relief.

Family History and Social History

Significant for a mother with headaches of an unknown type. The patient was married with 2 children, and worked as a homemaker.

Examination

Her cranial nerve screening was essentially within normal limits. There was a slight limitation in mouth opening (40 mm; normal, >45 mm), but the path of motion was symmetrical without deviation. There was no tenderness in the temporomandibular joint on palpation, and there was intermittent clicking upon opening widely. Functional testing, including chewing gum, did not cause pain. The cervical spine function was normal. A muscle palpation examination revealed some tenderness in the left anterior temporalis and left masseter muscles.

Behavioral Assessment

Unrevealing.

Discussion

This patient has a facial presentation of migraine without aura. Migraine must be differentiated from secondary headache disorders. The International Headache Society (IHS) has put forward specific criteria for headache classification, which include 13 major categories. Three are primary headache disorders (migraine, tension type, and cluster). The other 10 categories form the secondary headache class, where organic etiology is well defined.

Even though all pain in the head and face is conducted by the trigeminal nerve, the classification allows for clinical symptoms to be subclassified. This enables each classified entity to be studied, helping determine the pathophysiology and, ultimately, the treatment.

Lovshin was the first to describe migraine as a facial pain problem that could occur without pain in the first division of the trigeminal nerve. The pain in facial migraine is described as dull pain with superimposed throbbing, occurring once to several times per week. Each attack may last minutes to hours.

Raskin described ipsilatertal carotid tenderness in facial migraine, a finding also seen when migraine occurs in the head. This condition has also been referred to as *carotidynia*.

Treatment

Treatment of facial migraine is no different from that of more typical migraine presentations in the head. All management plans should include an understanding that the disorder is genetic, and that the goals should be to reduce pain frequency and intensity, restore function, and provide a sense of self-control.

Therapy may involve nonpharmacologic and pharmacologic approaches. In general, addressing triggering factors through diet, sleep, and exercise is part of first-line treatment.

The acute attack is treated early by administration of the most effective therapy. Analgesics, ergots, and triptans are most commonly used. If the migraines are painful and disabling, a triptan should be used as the first acute-care medication.

If the headaches are frequent, preventive medications may be considered. The groups of preventive medications most commonly used for migraine (including migraine with facial pain) are ß-blockers, calcium channel blockers, antidepressants, and antiepileptic drugs. Several other categories have been tried, and most medications (other than the Food and Drug Administration–approved methysergide, propranolol, timolol, and divalproex sodium) are used off label.

Second Diagnosis and Discussion

Headache may result from temporomandibular structures, as may pain in the temporomandibular joint (TMJ) be referred to as secondary to a primary headache diagnosis. Functional disorders and pain in the anatomic region of the TMJ and associated musculature are referred to as the *temporomandibular disorders (TMD)*.

This overlap between pain in the TMJ and true TMD is primarily related to the anatomy and neural innervations. It is essential not to confuse the issue and suggest a cause-and-effect relationship based on treatment responses. Because the trigeminal nerve is the final pathway for both head pain and TMD, the relationship between TMD and headache can be confusing. It is suggested that the 2 are separate, but may be aggravating or perpetuating factors for each other. Patients with primary headache can see their pain worsened or triggered when there is a coexisting TMD.

Epidemiology

TMD epidemiology has not specifically differentiated headache from facial pain. In non–patient population studies, 75% have at least 1 joint dysfunction sign (clicking, limited range of motion) and about 33% have at least 1 symptom (pain, pain on palpation). Of the 75% with 1 sign or symptom, fewer than 5% require treatment and even fewer have headache.

Etiology

Inflammation within the joint accounts for TMD pain, and the dysfunction is due to a disk or condyle incoordination. Muscle pain disorders may include spasm, myositis, muscle splinting, and myofascial pain.

The most frequent muscle disorder included in TMD classification is *myofascial pain.* Characteristically, myofascial pain is seen as pain and autonomic changes associated with tender areas in the muscle called *trigger points* (TPs). When palpated, these TPs produce a characteristic referred pain pattern.

Muscle tenderness is viewed by some clinicians as a potential cause of headache, although the cause–effect relation is still not clarified. Increased tenderness in pericranial muscles is the most prominent clinical finding in patients with tension-type headache and migraine. A hypothesis for myofascial pain requires a mechanical or chemical trauma to the muscle, which leads to sensitization of local peripheral nociceptors. This causes increased peripheral nociceptive input, leading to central sensitization at the spinal dorsal horn or trigeminal level. Once central sensitization has occurred, there can be retrograde referral to distant sites. The presence of silent pain receptors or nociceptors, a class of small-diameter nociceptors activated only after high-intensity peripheral stimulus, may account for the unusual referred patterns.

Other commonly suggested etiologic factors for headaches associated with TMD are bruxism, trauma, occlusal interferences, and emotional stressors. Many authors have reported a reduction in headache when they addressed treatment toward masticatory system functional disturbances. Because bruxism is so common a problem, it is hard to attribute its action to the pain etiology.

Although these oral parafunctional habits have been implicated in TMD, their relationship to headache remains unknown. Occlusal interferences are by far the most controversial aspect of etiology and treatment in TMD and related headache. Many studies suggest that changing the occlusion will eliminate headache. A literature meta-analysis does not support occlusion as a factor in headache etiology. Splint therapy is very effective in treating TMD, but it does not imply that the teeth are causal in the disorder.

Treatment of TMD

Patients with TMD are generally treated appropriately, with few long-term residual problems. It is reassuring to TMD patients that their problems are self-limiting and are rarely present beyond the fourth decade. Patients who are unresponsive to physical medicine approaches should not automatically be considered surgical candidates; rather, behavioral factors perpetuating the disorder should be considered.

In TMD/headache studies, there is little conformity in the headache treated, or even the outcome variable assessed, making the relationship difficult to gauge. Often there is the generalization that if treating the TMD decreases headache, the etiology must stem from the joint or muscle. The belief that all primary headaches are only generated peripherally does not fit with current knowledge describing pathogenesis of migraine. The peripheral therapies aimed at TMD may reduce headache, but care should be exercised in making a cause-and-effect determination when patients respond.

General management principles include decreasing pain, decreasing adverse loading (abnormal stresses on the TMJ), and restoring function. This

Table. Basic TMD Management Principles

1. Patient education and self-care

2. Cognitive behavioral interventions

3. Pharmacologic management
   (eg, analgesics, anti-inflammatories, muscle relaxants, sedatives, antidepressants)

4. Physical therapies
   (eg, posture training, stretching exercises, mobilization, physical modalities, appliance therapy, occlusal therapy)

5. Surgery
   (eg, arthrocentesis, arthroscopy, arthrotomy, and total joint replacement)

is best achieved through a structured, time-limited program addressing the physical disorder and its perpetuating factors. The 5 basic areas considered in TMD therapy are summarized in the Table.

It is believed that TMD is an aggravating factor in headache, and is only considered to be the cause if it is clearly related to clinical signs and symptoms involving the masticatory system. Until proof of headache mechanisms relating to TMD is available, the association may be coincidental. This should in no way deter clinicians from treating headache with proven therapies aimed at the temporomandibular structures; rather, it should caution drawing conclusions that if treatment is effective, then the cause is the TMD.

Further Comments on This Patient

In this patient, the IHS criteria for migraine without aura were met. The pain location and TMJ clicking were coincidental. Initially, the patient was asked to keep a daily diary to monitor the pain, medication use, and activity. She called 2 days later with severe pain, nausea, and light sensitivity.

She was brought to the office, where the examination results were unchanged. Sumatriptan (Imitrex) 6 mg SQ was administered, and the subject was observed. Within 30 minutes, the pain was gone.

After the pain frequency was tracked with the diary, it appeared the subject was having at least 2 episodes per week. A ß-blocker (nadolol 20 mg) was started at bedtime, and she was instructed to use a tablet of sumatriptan 50 mg at the onset of headache. The pain frequency lessened significantly, and the oral triptan proved very effective.

An explanation was given to the patient regarding the joint noise. No treatment was recommended. The patient was encouraged to exercise regularly, and other triggering factors were explored. After 12 months, she stopped the nadolol, and continues to have occasional pain that is controlled with sumatriptan.

Conclusion

Facial migraine is not common, but may be misdiagnosed as TMD. A careful history should always include questions that would help differentiate migraine from TMD. The presence of TMJ noise does not automatically suggest there is involvement. The diagnosis of a TMD should include 3 of the following 4 criteria: 1) joint noise; 2) joint tenderness; 3) limited range of motion; and 4) functional pain (ie, pain with chewing). If there is TMD in a patient with migraine, treatment may reduce the frequency of triggered headaches. In coexisting conditions, prophylaxis with a tricyclic antidepressant may be most beneficial.

Editors' Comment

Dr. Graff-Radford carefully reviews the necessary findings for TMD. Like other peripheral disorders, TMD may aggravate migraine in patients with biologic predisposition and is worthy of attention. Many headache patients have symptoms referable to the TMJ area, and a large percentage of them arrive at our center with the diagnosis of TMD. Most of the time, their previous treatment, directed at alleviating the TMD, has been unsuccessful, but treatment of their migraine symptoms is usually quite successful.

Diagnosis: Migraine With Facial Pain (Facial Migraine)

Selected Reading

Dworkin SF, LeResche LR, Von Korff M, et al. Epidemiology of signs and symptoms in temporomandibular disorders: 1. Clinical signs in cases and controls. *J Am Dent Assoc.* 1990;120:273-281.

Forssell H, Kirveskari P, Kangasniemi P. Distinguishing between headaches responsive and unresponsive to treatment of mandibular dysfunction. *Proc Finn Dent Soc.* 1986;82:219-222.

Gelb H, Tarte J. A two-year clinical dental evaluation of 200 cases of chronic headache: the cranio-cervical mandibular syndrome. *J Am Dent Assoc.* 1975;91:1230-1236.

Graff-Radford SB, Reeves JL, Jaeger B. Management of head and neck pain: effectiveness of altering factors perpetuating myofascial pain. *Headache.* 1987;27:186-190.

Jensen R, Bendtsen L, Olesen J. Muscular factors are important in tension-type headache. *Headache.* 1998;38:10-17.

Lovshin LL. Vascular neck pain—a common syndrome seldom recognized: analysis of 100 consecutive cases. *Cleve Clin Q.* 1960;27:5-13.

Magnusson T, Carlsson GE. Changes in recurrent headache and mandibular dysfunction after various types of dental treatment. *Acta Odont Scand.* 1980;38:311-320.

McNeill C, ed. *Craniomandibular Disorders: Guidelines for Evaluation, Diagnosis and Management.* 2nd ed. Chicago, Ill: Quintessence; 1992.

Mense S. Considerations concerning the neurobiological basis of muscle pain. *Can J Physiol Pharm.* 1991;9:610-616.

Mense S. Nociception from skeletal muscle in relation to clinical muscle pain. *Pain.* 1993; 54:241-289.

Raskin NH, Prusiner S. Carotidynia. *Neurology.* 1977;27:43-46.

Schiffman E, Fricton JR. Epidemiology of TMJ and craniofacial pain. In: Fricton JR, Kroening RJ, Hathaway KM, eds. *TMJ and Craniofacial Pain: Diagnosis and Management.* St. Louis, Mo: IEA Publishers; 1988:1-10.

Schiffman E, Fricton JR, Haley D, Shapiro BL. The prevalence and treatment needs of subjects with temporomandibular disorders. *J Am Dent Assoc.* 1989;120:295-304.

Seligman DA, Pullinger AG. The role of functional occlusal relationships in temporomandibular disorders. *J Craniomandib Disord Facial Oral Pain.* 1991;5:231-238.

Travell JG, Simons D. *Myofascial Pain and Dysfunction. The Trigger Point Manual.* Baltimore, Md: Williams and Wilkins; 1988.

11. The Child With Bad Headaches

A. David Rothner, MD

Director, Pediatric/Adolescent Headache Program
The Cleveland Clinic Foundation
Cleveland, Ohio

Case

RW, a 6-year-old girl, was evaluated for recurrent episodes of vomiting and headache.

As an infant, RW had experienced several unexplained episodes of irritability and vomiting, each lasting 2 to 3 hours. Trips to the pediatrician failed to reveal an etiology. At approximately age 3, she had several unexplained episodes of severe gait instability without loss of consciousness, each lasting a few minutes. These episodes disappeared spontaneously. Between ages 4 and 6, the girl had not experienced either of these types of episodes.

Approximately 3 months before presenting, RW had come home from preschool appearing very pale and quiet. Her eyes were glassy and were underlined by rings. On this occasion and during similar episodes, she had refused after-school snacks. The child wanted to be held by her mother and seemed to be bothered by light and noise. She cried and said that her head hurt.

These episodes lasted 20 to 30 minutes, followed by refusal to take water or food, occasional vomiting, and sleep lasting 2 to 3 hours. No coexisting infection or fever was noted.

When asked to describe the pain, RW said it felt like "a drum is hitting my head." When asked to point to the faces on a pain chart denoting severity, she reported the pain as being 8 out of 10. On closer questioning, there were no neurologic symptoms such as ataxia, weakness, visual impairment, and personality change.

Developmental History

RW was the product of a normal pregnancy, labor, and delivery. Her growth and development were normal.

Past Medical History

Medical history was negative for any serious illnesses or allergies.

Review of Systems

System review revealed no medical problems of note. RW was intellectually and developmentally normal, and behavioral issues were denied.

Family History

There was a positive family history for episodic headaches in the mother and maternal grandmother.

Exam

RW's general physical examination produced entirely normal results. Her neurologic findings (including gait), cranial nerves (including visual fields and fundi), motor examination, and cerebellar testing were normal.

Treatment Course

An initial diagnosis of migraine was made. At the time of diagnosis, the youngster was having 1 or 2 episodes per month, and it was felt that symptomatic management would be appropriate.

The following suggestions were made: At the onset of the headache, the youngster should be taken to a dark, quiet, cool room. A cold compress should be applied to the forehead and kept there with a headband. The youngster should be offered small sips of water, if tolerated. She should be given 10 mg/kg liquid ibuprofen, as well as a teaspoon of diphenhydramine (Benadryl), and allowed to fall asleep.

The mother called back approximately 6 weeks later and stated that some of the episodes were now accompanied by severe vomiting and that the medication would not stay down. She was instructed that should the vomiting occur within 30 minutes of administration of the medicine or should the medicine be visible in the vomitus, the medication should be repeated. Trimethobenzamide 100 mg was prescribed in a suppository form, to be given at the onset of the attack to decrease the nausea and vomiting.

Approximately 3 months later, RW was re-evaluated. The girl's attacks had increased in frequency and duration. The attacks were now always associated with nausea and vomiting, lasted 3 to 4 hours, and occurred once a week. There were no symptoms of increased intracranial pressure or progressive neurologic disease, and she had a completely normal re-examination.

The pros and cons of various preventive medications were discussed with RW's mother, even though they were not approved for prevention of migraine in children. Because of her age, cyproheptadine was considered the medication of choice. RW was started on 1 teaspoon (2 mg) of cyproheptadine every night for 2 weeks. It was explained to her mother that potential side effects included lethargy and increased appetite.

After 2 weeks on this dosage, RW tolerated the medication well, and the dose was increased to 2 teaspoons at night. Four weeks later, the mother reported that the spells were significantly decreased in frequency and severity. Two months later, they had disappeared entirely; 2 months after that, the medication was discontinued. One year later, RW experiences only mild, intermittent spells.

Discussion

Roughly 20% of pediatric primary care patients have recurrent headache. In patients younger than age 7, the majority of these headaches are migraine. Most of these children never report the problem to their physician.

These headaches can affect the lifestyle of both the child and his or her family, and, when severe, can lead to time lost from school and extracurricular activities, as well as time lost from work by the parents. The majority of headaches seen in young children are related to infections or minor trauma.

Only a very small percentage have serious life-threatening disorders, which usually can be identified from accompanying symptoms and signs. Careful history can usually help pinpoint the type of headache and its cause.

The prevalence of all types of headaches is 3% to 8% at 3 years, 20% at 5 years, and 37% to 52% at 7 years. The incidence rises to 57% to 82% from ages 7 to 15. Approximately 1% to 3% of 7-year-olds and 4% to 11% of 7- to 15-year-olds experience migraine headaches. Before puberty, boys and girls are affected equally; after puberty, migraine is more common in girls. At times, these migraine headaches can be associated with an occasional tension-type headache.

Migraines are acute recurrent headaches. They are not daily. They are painful but not life-threatening, and often are accompanied by anorexia, nausea, or vomiting. If neurologic symptoms or signs accompany the migraine headache, an underlying neurologic reason should be sought.

The pathogenesis of migraine in children is the same as in adults and is discussed elsewhere in this book. The most frequently encountered form of migraine is "common migraine," now called "migraine without aura." There are no associated neurologic features. The general physical and neurologic examinations are entirely normal. Laboratory and imaging are not necessary when patients have "straightforward" migraine. Further testing is only needed if the child is critically ill or the history or physical examination suggests a neurologic disorder.

Approximately 15% of children with migraine have migraine with aura. In most instances, the headaches are episodic and paroxysmal, not daily, and are often precipitated by triggers such as anxiety, stress, fatigue, lack of sleep, minor head injury, exercise, travel, and illness. At times, dietary factors are important.

Migraine is a familial disorder, but the mode of inheritance is not clear. Positive family history of migraine is reported in 70% to 80% of youngsters.

There are numerous other forms of migraine that present in children. The old term, "complex migraine," describes migraine associated with neurologic deficits, including hemiplegia with weakness on one side. Ophthalmoplegic migraine is characterized by dilation of one pupil and drooping of the eyelid. Basilar artery migraine generally consists of occipital headache associated with balance difficulty and dizziness, while confusional migraine is associated with inability to understand or communicate appropriately. All require neurologic evaluation.

Migraine variants include conditions such as episodic torticollis, cyclic vomiting, paroxysmal vertigo, and the "Alice in Wonderland syndrome"—in which the patient sees very small (micropsia) or large distortions (macropsia) during aura. These conditions require additional evaluation.

Treatment

Once a diagnosis of migraine is made, the next step is patient–parent education and formulation of a treatment plan. If the attacks are brief and easily relieved by sleep, minimal or no medication may be indicated. For children whose attacks are of a longer duration, episodic, symptomatic therapy is sufficient. For children experiencing frequent, severe, and/or prolonged attacks, a combination of symptomatic and preventive medication should be utilized.

The patient and parents should be instructed to keep a headache calendar and to recognize triggers or precipitating factors so that they can be reduced or eliminated. Nonpharmacologic measures such as stress reduction and biofeedback may be beneficial.

The mainstay of symptomatic treatment is intermittent oral analgesics (Table). The nonsteroidal anti-inflammatory drugs (NSAIDs) seem to be more effective than acetaminophen. For more severe attacks, they can be used together. These agents should be taken at maximum doses at the onset of the headache.

The dose recommendation for ibuprofen is 10 mg/kg; in the case of acetaminophen, it is 15 mg/kg. The liquid formulations seem to be better tol-

Table. Treatment of Pediatric Migraine Headaches

Therapy and Medication	Dosage	Comments
Symptomatic:		
Acetaminophen	10-15 mg/kg q 4-6 h	Available as suppository
Ibuprofen	4-10 mg/kg q 6-8 h	No suppository available
Trimethobenzamide HCl	15-20 mg/kg, divided q 6 h	Antiemetic; available as 100- or 200-mg suppository
Diphenhydramine (Benadryl)	25-50 mg	Sedative
Preventive:		
Amitriptyline HCl	0.1-2.0 mg/kg hs	Cardiac conduction problems possible; anticholinergic side effects
Cyproheptadine HCl (Periactin)	0.25 mg/kg	Side effects include sedation and increased appetite
Propranolol (HCl) (Inderal)	0.6-1.5 mg/kg, in 3 divided doses	Cardiac complications possible; side effects include vivid dreams and depression
Valproic acid (Depakote)	10-30 mg/kg, in 2-3 divided doses	Hepatic or pancreatic dysfunction possible; side effects include anorexia and weight gain
Verapamil HCl (Calan, Isoptin)	4-8 mg/kg, in 3 divided doses	Side effects include constipation, sedation, weight gain, depression

erated and more rapidly absorbed. Medications containing barbiturates, opiates, or caffeine should be avoided.

Antiemetics can be helpful in reducing nausea and vomiting. Sleep often relieves headaches, and sedatives such as diphenhydramine may be useful. Abortive medications such as the triptans are not currently approved for children younger than age 18 and are not generally recommended as first-line therapy. Some pediatric neurologists use them successfully for intractable patients, especially in children whose headaches have not responded to conventional OTC medications and whose attacks are of a long duration and disabling.

Preventive treatment may be indicated for patients with severe, frequent, or prolonged migraine that interferes with normal social activities or has not responded adequately to symptomatic treatment (Table). Preventive medication is also appropriate for children using OTC medications more than 2 or 3 times per week. No preventive migraine medications are approved by the FDA for this age group; however, ß-blockers, calcium channel blockers, NSAIDs, tricyclic antidepressants, cyproheptadine, and anticonvulsants have all been used. In younger children, cyproheptadine can be quite helpful, but it should not be used in obese children.

Although ß-blockers may be useful, care should be taken in using this category of medication in children with bronchospastic disease, diabetes mellitus, or Wolff-Parkinson-White syndrome. Side effects may include fatigue, depression, and sleep problems, as well as decreased athletic endurance. Very few data are available on the efficacy of calcium channel blockers and anticonvulsants in this age group.

Tricyclic antidepressants have been used in children and adolescents for many conditions, ranging from enuresis to migraine. Some patients cannot tolerate the anticholinergic side effects such as dry mouth, blurred vision, urinary retention, and constipation. The usual dosage of amitriptyline is 0.1 to 1 mg/kg, given at bedtime. It should be started in low doses and slowly increased so that the patient "adjusts" to the side effects.

Nonpharmacologic techniques for reducing headache include sleep hygiene, diet modification, and exercise. Biofeedback has been demonstrated to be effective.

The short-term outlook for children with migraine is favorable. More than half the patients show improvement within 6 months with or without medical intervention, and approximately two-thirds experience remission for 2 or more years during adolescence. More than half of individuals who have migraines as children will continue to have attacks in adulthood.

Editors' Note

There are several important issues for diagnosis and treatment of children with migraine. From a diagnostic standpoint, pediatric migraine is of a shorter duration and more frequently bilateral than that in adults, with early onset of more severe nausea and vomiting. Sleep interrupts and aborts the attacks more frequently, and often the pain attacks are less severe. Migraine variants are more common, including vertigo, cyclical vomiting, abdominal pain, and motion sickness.

Proving efficacy with triptans compared to placebo has been difficult in children, because the attacks are short-lived, and pediatric patients respond more readily to treatment, resulting in high placebo responses. No oral triptan has been found to be statistically superior to placebo in children.

Sumatriptan (Imitrex) nasal spray has been found to be superior to placebo in 5 international trials, and has already received regulatory approval in some countries. Long-term safety was also established for sumatriptan nasal spray in adolescents in an extension trial.

A nasal spray should be optimal for children, as this formulation addresses the quick onset and rapid escalation of pain, the short attack duration, and the high incidence of nausea and vomiting in the pediatric population. In addition, the orally dissolving tablets are also a preferred formulation for younger children, as they are easy to administer and the child does not have to swallow a tablet with liquid.

At the New England Center for Headache, we also treat most children with headache with biofeedback training and other behavioral methods, vitamins, and minerals before considering the stronger acute care and preventive medications.

<u>Diagnosis:</u> Pediatric Migraine Without Aura

Selected Reading

Guidetti V, Russell G, Sillanpää M, Winner P, eds. *Headache and Migraine in Childhood and Adolescence.* London: Martin Dunitz; 2002.

Rothner AD. Primary care and management of headache in children and adolescents. *Fam Pract Recert.* 2002;24:29-45.

Wasiewski WW, Rothner AD. Pediatric migraine headache: diagnosis, evaluation and management. *The Neurologist.* 1999;5:122-134.

Winner P, Rothner AD, eds. *Headache in Children and Adolescents.* Hamilton, Ontario: BC Decker; 2001.

12. The Woman With Headache During Pregnancy

Elizabeth Loder, MD, FACP

Director, Headache and Pain Management Programs
Spaulding Rehabilitation Hospital
Boston, Massachusetts

Case

A 38-year-old woman in the 17th week of her third pregnancy was referred by her obstetrician-gynecologist for consultation. The patient had a 16-year history of migraine without aura. For several years, she had used sumatriptan (Imitrex) 50 mg PO to treat individual headaches. This provided complete relief of 60% of the attacks and partial relief for the remainder of the attacks. She occasionally required a second dose, but had no significant side effects resulting from the medication.

Despite this good response to abortive treatment, the frequency of headaches at times required prophylactic treatment. For 18 months before conception, the patient had been maintained on sodium valproate (Depakote), with a reduction in headache frequency from 8 to 4 attacks per month. The sodium valproate was discontinued when her pregnancy was confirmed, and she was advised to discontinue the use of sumatriptan.

Headache frequency and severity increased after discontinuation of the patient's usual treatment regimen. However, the patient was highly motivated to avoid medication use during her first trimester. Both she and her obstetrician expected that headaches would abate after the first trimester of pregnancy was completed. However, that did not occur.

At the time of referral, the patient was experiencing 2 headaches per week on average, each lasting up to 2 days. They were unilateral headaches, associated with nausea and prolonged vomiting, photophobia, and exacerbation with physical activity.

She has been treated symptomatically with prochlorperazine suppositories and an oral acetaminophen–oxycodone preparation. Although this provided some relief, the patient reported significant difficulty in caring for her 2 young children.

Family History

Significant for mother with migraines, which did not resolve during pregnancies.

Past Medical History and Review of Systems

Completely normal and healthy.

General and Neurologic Exam

Normal.

Discussion

Migraine affects at least 16% of American women. Prevalence is highest during the childbearing years, with the result that migraine and pregnancy will commonly coexist. This case illustrates a number of important points about the presentation and treatment of migraine in pregnancy.

First, not all women with migraine will experience relief of headache during pregnancy. Although retrospective studies have suggested that more than one half of migraineurs experience headache remission with pregnancy, a prospective study by Scharff and colleagues suggests that only one third resolve. It further shows that if headaches are a problem at the end of the first trimester, they are likely to continue to be a problem throughout the remainder of the pregnancy.

There is some reason to believe that women whose prepregnancy headaches were correlated with hormonal fluctuations such as menstruation are more likely to experience headache resolution with the stable hormonal levels of pregnancy. In addition, women who suffer from migraine with aura may be less likely to experience reduction in headache frequency as a result of pregnancy.

The patient in this case was well into her second trimester and continued to experience severe, disabling headaches. She required treatment beyond reassurance and symptomatic medication.

Second, it is vitally important to anticipate, rather than react to, the possibility of pregnancy in any migraine patient of childbearing potential. Ideally, a pregnancy would be planned, and steps to minimize drug exposures and optimize nonpharmacologic treatment strategies would be taken before conception. In reality, 50% of pregnancies in the United States are unintended, so it is not uncommon for women undergoing migraine treatment to unexpectedly become pregnant, often while on a variety of medications.

Inadvertent fetal exposure to headache medications in this situation can generate a great deal of anxiety. Patients with pregnancy exposures to medication can seek information from one of several national teratogen information services (www.gsk.com for sumatriptan and naratriptan; 1-800-236-9933 for zolmitriptan; 1-800-986-8999 for rizatriptan; 1-888-233-2334 for sodium valproate).

It is especially desirable to avoid medication use during the first trimester, when most organogenesis occurs. This patient was taking a medication (sodium valproate) that is a known teratogen, associated with roughly a 1% to 2% risk of neural tube defects in exposed fetuses. The neural tube forms at day 28, so in assessing the risk to this patient's pregnancy, it will be important to establish the timing of conception and medication discontinuation. Serum α-fetoprotein levels and ultrasound evaluation can also be used to screen for neural tube pathology. However, it would clearly be better to have warned the patient about the need to avoid pregnancy at the time of sodium valproate prescription.

Third, nonpharmacologic, behavioral, and physical techniques should be emphasized in the management of headache occurring in pregnancy. Biofeedback, physical therapy, trigger point injections, and relaxation techniques can all be useful.

In one study, pregnant patients treated with physical therapy, relaxation, and biofeedback had an 81% reduction in headache, compared to a 33% reduction in a control population. Third-party payers, who generally do not provide coverage for these methods of treatment, will often approve exceptions for pregnant patients, in an effort to avert medication use.

In women with identifiable trigger points, local anesthetic infiltration can be safely performed during pregnancy. All of these methods should be considered for use in the case patient. Even if they are incompletely effective, they may provide important augmentative benefits to other therapy.

"Avoidance therapy," involving the identification and elimination of headache trigger factors (eg, excess caffeine, lack of sleep, or skipping of meals), should be emphasized. A temporary reduction in work hours or a medical leave of absence from work may also be useful in avoiding the need for pharmacologic treatment of headaches. If effective, such strategies are clearly preferable to pharmacologic treatment of headache during pregnancy. With 2 young children and a job, the patient may benefit from a reduction in work hours, assignment to less taxing duties, or obtaining household or family help with home and child care responsibilities.

The use of herbs, vitamins, and dietary supplements to treat migraine in pregnancy should be discouraged. Although commonly perceived to be "natural" and, therefore, safe, most such preparations have not been thoroughly studied in pregnancy. Some, such as feverfew, which affects platelet aggregability, are potentially dangerous.

Fourth, drug treatment of migraine headache is largely based on expert consensus and is empiric. Women of childbearing potential are usually excluded from drug studies or are required to take strict precautions against pregnancy, leading to a lack of evidence upon which to base treatment recommendations.

The FDA rates drugs for use in pregnancy using a 5-category scale. Drugs in category A are those for which controlled studies fail to show risk; in category B, animal studies do not suggest the possibility of adverse effects; in category C, it is difficult to assess risk and it is suggested that the physician and patient weigh the risk-to-benefit ratio carefully; in category D, there is positive evidence suggestive of risk to human fetuses; and in category X, risk in pregnancy is judged to be unacceptable. The FDA ratings for drugs commonly used to treat migraine in pregnancy are listed in the Table (page 90).

This patient's current abortive regimen of a phenothiazine antiemetic and an opioid in combination with acetaminophen is recommended by many experts. Both drugs have a reassuring track record for use over time in pregnancy. However, they are less effective than specific migraine medications (ie, the triptans), and have undesirable side effects, including sedation, constipation, and the potential to be habit-forming, that make their use problematic in some women.

The use of triptans is not recommended during pregnancy. Results of a prospective pregnancy registry, along with 2 large Scandinavian retrospective studies of sumatriptan use in pregnancy, have ruled out the possibility of a very large increase in teratogenic risk because of first-trimester exposure. However, very large numbers of exposed pregnancies are necessary to rule out smaller increases in risk or to provide conclusive evidence of safety. This makes a positive recommendation for use in pregnancy inadvisable. These results are very reassuring, however, for women who have had unplanned exposure in pregnancy.

Fifth, in some women with severe or disabling migraine, the benefits of prophylactic treatment may be judged to outweigh the risks. This is particularly true in patients who experience severe headaches in association with prolonged vomiting and dehydration.

In these cases of severe prostration, common sense suggests that untreated headache and its consequences, as well as use of unsupervised medications by a desperate patient, may be more dangerous than a traditional prophylactic treatment regimen. Medications selected for use should be those that, based on current knowledge, are least likely to pose a danger to mother or fetus.

In the case of migraine prophylactic drugs, those with which we have the largest experience of use for other conditions are ß-blockers and tricyclic antidepressants. The lowest possible dose of the drug necessary to produce acceptable improvement should be used. Drugs such as anticonvulsants (especially sodium valproate), methysergide (Sansert), and lithium should be avoided, as safer treatment choices exist.

The patient in this case should first be treated with nonpharmacologic strategies. However, if disabling headaches continue, she may be a candidate for prophylaxis with a ß-blocker or tricyclic antidepressant.

Before any treatment for migraine is prescribed for a pregnant patient, it is important to review with the patient that the risk of fetal malformation is 2% to 4%, even in the absence of any medication use. Absolute guarantees about the safety of a regimen should not be made; rather, the patient and physician should carefully assess the risks and benefits of treatment alternatives.

Other important issues concerning migraine and pregnancy are not specifically suggested by this case, but nonetheless should be raised. The first is

Table. FDA Pregnancy Ratings for Commonly Used Migraine Medications

Drug	U.S. Food and Drug Administration Pregnancy Rating
All triptans	C
Aspirin	C
Butalbital	C
Codeine	B
Acetaminophen	B
Butorphanol	B

B, animal studies do not suggest the possibility of adverse effects; C, it is difficult to assess the risk; it is suggested that the physician and patient weigh the risk-to-benefit ratio carefully.

that migraine does not appear to be correlated with poor pregnancy outcomes. That is, there is no reason to believe that migraine itself increases the risk of either pregnancy complications or the occurrence of birth defects.

A second issue is that, in addition to changes in pre-existing headache, conditions that can be provoked by pregnancy (migraine, particularly migraine with aura) can occur for the first time during pregnancy or after delivery. Evaluation of new or worsening headaches in the pregnant patient should be as thorough as that in nonpregnant patients, including imaging studies if deemed necessary.

Some secondary causes of headache are more likely to occur during pregnancy, including subarachnoid hemorrhage and cerebral venous thrombosis; moreover, some headaches are related to pregnancy-specific conditions. In pre-eclampsia, headache and other vague complaints can occur well before objective signs of the disorder, such as hypertension and proteinuria, are discovered. Whether pre-eclampsia is more likely to occur in migraineurs has not been definitely determined. A history of recurrent spontaneous abortions or thromboembolic disease in combination with migraine-like headaches should suggest the possibility of antiphospholipid antibody syndrome.

Third, once this patient's pregnancy is completed, her plans for future birth control should be ascertained. Some women with migraine experience worsening of headache with oral contraceptives and will need to use alternative methods. In addition, there is controversy concerning the use of oral contraceptives in women with migraine, based on the elevated risk of ischemic stroke associated with both migraine (especially migraine with aura) and oral contraceptives. The new lower-dose estrogen pills may be less likely to worsen migraine, and also seem to be associated with a lower risk of ischemic stroke.

Fourth, because it provides important health benefits for mother and child, our patient should be encouraged to breast-feed. Unfortunately, evidence shows that lactation does not protect against migraine, even though regular breast-feeding can delay the return of hormonal cycles and theoretically might be expected to have a beneficial impact on the migraine patient.

Less than 4% of a 6-mg parenteral maternal dose of sumatriptan is excreted into breast milk, and none of the drug can be recovered in the milk after 8 hours. Therefore, many physicians allow patients to use a triptan during lactation, but recommend that they pump and discard their breast milk for 8 hours after use. Sumatriptan, with its short half-life (2 hours), may have an advantage in this situation, as it almost completely gone from the body in 10 hours.

Fifth, depression and other affective disorders are highly comorbid with migraine. The occurrence of depression during pregnancy, postpartum depression, and milder forms of postpartum affective illness such as the "baby blues" may be more likely to occur in migraineurs, and should be carefully monitored.

With attention to detail and careful planning, even migraineurs with severe illness can experience reasonable headache control during pregnancy. There is thus no reason for migraineurs to avoid or postpone pregnancy because of their illness.

Editors' Note

This excellent review by Dr. Loder gives many facts and pearls about treating the pregnant migraineur. We strongly encourage biofeedback and other behavioral and physical techniques, as well as permitting our patients to take vitamin B_2 and magnesium after speaking to their obstetrician. We also withhold herbs and almost any acute care medications, including aspirin, butalbital combinations, and triptans. On rare occasions, we will permit opiates and even steroids, which obstetricians use frequently in certain situations.

<u>Diagnosis:</u> Migraine Without Aura in Pregnancy

Selected Reading

Scharff L, Marcus DA, Turk DC. Headache during pregnancy and in the postpartum: a prospective study. *Headache.* 1997;37:203-210.

Scharff L, Marcus DA, Turk DC. Maintenance of effects in the nonmedical treatment of headaches during pregnancy. *Headache.* 1996;36:285-290.

Shuhaiber S, Pastuszak A, Schick B, et al. Pregnancy outcome following first trimester exposure to sumatriptan. *Neurology.* 1998;51:581-583.

Wood A. Drugs in pregnancy. *N Engl J Med.* 2000;338:1130-1137.

13. Headache and Neck Pain After Trauma to the Head

Joel R. Saper, MD, FACP, FAAN

Director and Founder, Michigan Head Pain and Neurological Institute
Director and Founder, Head Pain Treatment Program, Chelsea Community Hospital
Professor (Clinical) of Medicine (Neurology)
Michigan State University
Ann Arbor, Michigan

Case

A 25-year-old man complains of daily headache that began after head trauma.

The man was involved in a motor vehicle accident in which he was struck from behind by a vehicle traveling approximately 15 to 20 mph when his car was stationary. His right parietal cranium struck the doorframe, but no loss of consciousness occurred. The patient felt dazed and within moments experienced a constant, right occipito-cervical pain associated with neck stiffness and limitation of motion. Eventually, the pain generalized to the entire cranium.

His pain was constant, occasionally throbbing, and sometimes associated with nausea and light sensitivity. Neck movement aggravated the headache as well as the neck pain, which remained right-sided. The patient was unable to return to work because movement aggravated his symptoms.

Visits to a series of physicians produced varying diagnoses, including post-traumatic headache, whiplash, and myofascial pain. A computed tomography scan of the head and magnetic resonance imaging of the cervical spine revealed no recognizable pathology. Analgesics, triptans, and tricyclic antidepressants provided only modest pain relief. Physical therapy increased the pain. A series of occipital nerve blocks resulted in transient, partial relief. During the course of the next year, the patient took increasing amounts of over-the-counter (OTC) analgesics and, eventually, opioid analgesics.

One year after the traumatic event, the patient was referred to a tertiary center. At that time he was using 8 to 10 mixed analgesics containing caffeine, aspirin, and acetaminophen daily; 1 to 2 rizatriptan tablets daily; and 10 to 12 oxycodone and acetaminophen tablets daily. In addition to daily and increasingly severe head and neck pain, the patient reported mild to moderate cognitive impairment, difficulty sleeping, and growing depression.

Past Medical History

Noncontributory.

Examination

Neurologic examination revealed a withdrawn young man appearing depressed and slow to respond. Speech was mildly slurred. Results of general neurologic examination were normal, except for mild dysarthria; otherwise, there was no impairment of cranial nerve or other motor or sensory systems. Examination of the cervico-occipital junction revealed bilateral tenderness. Examination of the facet joints demonstrated right-sided pain on manual manipulation. Limitation of motion and guarding were apparent. Bilateral tenderness was present in the trapezius muscles.

Course of Illness

Because attempts to treat the patient aggressively and reduce the need for analgesics had been without success while in the outpatient setting, he was admitted to a specialized inpatient facility. Rapid detoxification from medications was scheduled simultaneously with serial intravenous protocols, and involved the use of dihydroergotamine, chlorpromazine, diphenhydramine, ketorolac, and valproic acid. Moderate withdrawal symptoms were treated with oral clonazepam and prn tizanidine (Zanaflex). Neurocognitive impairment was assessed and considered drug- and pain-related. Indeed, the patient's dysarthria responded to detoxification.

Headache symptoms diminished from severe to moderate over the course of 5 days, but neck pain persisted. Diagnostic right cervical facet blockade at C2-C3 was undertaken with fluoroscopic control. Complete but transient relief was noted for 2 to 3 days. A second set of confirmatory facet blocks was undertaken, with similar transient, complete relief.

The patient was discharged from the hospital with a preventive program consisting of nadolol 40 mg bid, nortriptyline 75 mg hs, tizanidine 2-4 mg tid prn, and naproxen sodium 550 mg bid prn. Rizatriptan (Maxalt) tablets were used for acute migrainous events and restricted to 2 usage days per week.

One week after discharge, the patient underwent radiofrequency ablation of the right C2-C3 facet nerves. Two weeks after the procedure, the patient reported 90% reduction of neck pain and 80% reduction of daily headache from pretreatment levels. Depression was relieved substantially with the tricyclic agent, and rehabilitational efforts for return to work were instituted.

Discussion

Several plausible mechanisms for chronic posttraumatic headache exist. Soft tissue and mechanical injury to the cervico-occipital junction is generally accepted as causing at least acute cervical pain. Bogduk and associates have demonstrated a probable link between flexion–extension injury and headache.

Bartsch and Goadsby have demonstrated a direct influence on second- and third-order neurons in the trigeminal nucleus caudalis after stimulation at the C2-C3 level. Descending trigeminal pathways and inhibitory influences from the brain stem are physiologically intermingled with afferent systems from the occipitocervical junction and upper cervical spine. The increasingly understood nociceptive phenomena, the identified changes in wide dynamic neuronal function, and the phenomena of "windup" and "kindling" in the spinal cord and brain stem might well combine to form a plausible explanation for the transition from acute injury to chronic head and neck pain, and perhaps centrally maintained pain as well.

The periaqueductal gray region of the upper brain stem, and the location of the dorsal raphe nucleus and related areas, is currently cited as the vicinity of the migraine "generator." This area is intimately involved in pain modulation and is prone to injury from traumatic events.

Treatment

This patient demonstrated several important and therapeutically targetable phenomena. It is likely that he suffered from posttraumatic cephalalgia and cervical facet syndrome occurring as the result of a rear-end motor vehicle accident. His headaches appear to be a combination of posttraumatic migrainous cephalalgia aggravated by analgesic and triptan rebound and post-traumatic cervicalgia. Detoxification and treatments directed at his posttraumatic headaches appeared to provide moderate relief. Neck pain did not respond to this treatment, and required targeted therapeutic intervention.

It is likely that cervical pathology and nociceptive stimulation to the C2-3 level served to provoke and maintain the headache mechanism, and upon its termination, after facet radiofrequency ablation, the headache response improved dramatically. Depression resolved simultaneously with pain control. This may have been the result of antidepressant therapy or, more likely, due to a reduction of pain. Neurocognitive impairment seemed relieved after detoxification and pain control.

Conclusion

In the case described, a comprehensive approach to treatment was required, involving detoxification, central (migrainous) pain control, and treatment of cervicalgia, as well as addressing functions of emotional and rehabilitative concern.

Editors' Note

Dr. Saper and his colleagues at the Michigan Head Pain and Neurological Institute have accumulated years of experience in treating these very challenging patients. The editors believe the days of viewing this disorder as "psychological" or as driven by financial gain should be put behind us. Dr. Saper puts into sharp focus the role of cervical structures in this disorder and the necessity of an expert comprehensive approach.

<u>Diagnosis:</u> Chronic Post-traumatic Headache

Suggested Reading

Bartsch T, Goadsby PJ. Stimulation of the greater occipital nerve (GON) enhances responses of dural responsive convergent neurons in the trigeminal cervical complex in the rat. *Cephalalgia.* 2001;21:401-402.

Bogduk N. Headache and the neck. In: Goadsby PJ, Silberstein SD, eds. *Headache.* Boston, Mass: Butterworth-Heinemann; 1997:369-381.

Lord SM, Barnsley L, Wallis BJ, McDonald GJ, Bogduk N. Percutaneous radiofrequency neurotomy for chronic cervical zygapophyseal joint pain. *N Engl J Med.* 1996;335:1721-1726.

Saper JR. Chronic daily headache. *Headache* (in press).

Saper JR. Post-traumatic headache: a neurobehavioral disorder. *Arch Neurol.* 2000;57: 1776-1777.

Saper JR, Silberstein SD, Gordon CD, eds. *Handbook of Headache Management.* 2nd ed. Baltimore, Md: Lippincott Williams & Wilkins; 1999.

Wallis BJ, Lord SM, Bogduk N. Resolution of psychological distress of whiplash patients following treatment by radiofrequency neurotomy: a randomized, double-blind, placebo-controlled trial. *Pain.* 1997;73:15-22.

Weiller C, May A, Limmroth V, et al. Brainstem activation in human migraine attacks. *Nat Med.* 1995;1:858-860.

14. The Women With Headaches, Syncope, and Neurologic Features

Mark Stillman, MD

Headache and Pain Section
Department of Neurology
Cleveland Clinic Foundation
Cleveland, Ohio

Case 1

A 37-year-old female software engineer had a history of intermittent headaches dating back to her teens. She came to the clinic complaining of daily or near-daily headaches.

The headaches were characterized as bilateral, occipital, throbbing headaches of moderate to severe intensity. They were aggravated by routine physical activity and were associated with nausea, vomiting, photophobia, and osmophobia, but no phonophobia.

Before most of her headaches, the subject would develop a central white expanding scotoma surrounded by sparkling vision, lasting one-half hour to 1 hour. Periodically accompanying this were confusion, lightheadedness, and diplopia.

In the preceding year, the woman had experienced 6 episodes of syncope lasting more than 1 hour. The syncope would accompany an episode of light-headedness and confusion. For the previous 2 to 3 months, the subject had spent two thirds of the time with a headache. She had refrained from driving for fear of "blacking out" at the wheel.

Medications used by this patient included sertraline (Zoloft) 400 mg a day and trazodone 150 mg a night for depression and insomnia, respectively. While she used to rely on over-the-counter (OTC) analgesics for pain relief, the subject had stopped several months earlier because of lack of effect.

Family History

Significant for migraine in a sister and their mother.

Social History and Review of Systems

Unrevealing.

General Examination, Including Neurologic Examination

Normal.

Diagnostic Workup

Negative. Specifically, thyroid functions were normal, and there was no anemia, elevation in the sedimentation rate, or electrocardiogram abnormality. A magnetic resonance (MR) image of the brain, MR of the circle of Willis, MR venogram, and contrast study failed to demonstrate any abnormalities.

The patient was referred to the cardiac laboratory for evaluation of her episodes of syncope and had an extensive workup, including a heads-up tilt table (HUT) test, isoproterenol challenge test, radionuclide blood volume test, and a stress echocardiogram. This revealed postural orthostatic tachycardia syndrome (POTS) and cardioinhibitory syncope (vasovagal response).

Past Medication History

At the suggestion of the cardiologist, the subject was started on a low-dose ß-blocker. At 8-week follow-up, light-headedness and syncope had resolved, but headaches persisted at the same frequency, though at a lesser severity. Divalproex sodium was prescribed preventively, along with meto-clopramide and diclofenac to abort headaches. Ergot alkaloids and triptans have been avoided as abortive agents in this particular case.

Case 2

A 52-year-old woman referred herself to a tertiary-care headache clinic with an undiagnosed headache syndrome.

The patient had been seen by a number of physicians, including a senior neurologist, over the previous year, and had been labeled hysterical. She had a long history of headaches dating back to age 15, but the characteristics had recently changed.

After a bout of acute bronchitis 10 years earlier, the subject developed headaches accompanied by hand and leg tremors, leg weakness, and falls. She described dizziness, visual obscuration in both eyes and her whole visual field, and flashing bright lights. Her husband reported that the subject would develop confusion and incoherence lasting minutes. These spells occurred at least twice a week and were always accompanied by a headache. The subject had suffered 2 syncopal episodes in 12 months, but could not remember whether these had been linked specifically to headaches.

The headaches were described as throbbing, bilateral, occipital, or frontal. They were rated moderate to severe, were most severe perimenstrually, and were exacerbated by activity.

At another hospital, the woman was diagnosed as having migraine and placed on rizatriptan (Maxalt), trazodone, venlafaxine (Effexor), and clonaz-epam; in addition, she self-medicated with OTC combination headache reme-dies (8 tablets per week). At our institution on a previous occasion, she was felt to have a conversion reaction, and was sent for formal neuropsychologi-cal testing. This demonstrated high average intelligence without defects in higher cortical functioning. However, there was a mild to moderate rise in depression indices, consistent with depression. A semistructured psycho-logical interview confirmed somatic preoccupation and a pattern of non-restorative sleep with diffuse pains and aches.

Past Medical History

Significant for irritable bowel syndrome and a remote history of thyroid disease.

Family History
Strongly positive for migraine in mother, sisters, and daughter.

Social History
Noncontributory.

Examination
Normal.

Diagnostic Workup
Laboratory workup, including a thyroid panel, was unrevealing. Magnetic resonance imaging of the brain, with and without contrast, and MR venography/angiography were normal.

Referral to the cardiology syncope laboratory resulted in an extensive evaluation, including a HUT test. The test was truncated in the 38th minute, at 70 degrees' tilt, when the patient experienced light-headedness and tachycardia to 110 per minute; this was followed by a delayed drop in diastolic and systolic blood pressure. With resumption of the supine position, the hemodynamic abnormalities normalized. Blood volume testing was normal.

Past Medication History
The patient was previously prescribed low-dose propranolol, venlafaxine, and topiramate (Topamax). To abort headaches, she was prescribed indomethacin and metoclopramide.

At 8-week follow-up, the subject no longer complained of frequent headaches; every 2 to 3 weeks, she had a single headache that could be easily aborted. However, she still complained of episodes of light-headedness and visual blurring. Midodrine (ProAmatine) was recently added to treat the orthostasis of POTS.

Discussion
Basilar migraine, known formerly as basilar artery migraine, Bickerstaff's migraine, or syncopal migraine, is perhaps the most poorly understood of all readily recognizable headache disorders. First described in detail just 40 years ago, these enigmatic headaches have been the subject of very few authoritative studies; many of these were written in the pre–magnetic resonance imaging or early computed tomography era.

New research techniques and recent clinical observations have led to a resurgence of interest in basilar migraine, and these headaches may be more common than previously thought. As will be described below, clinical recognition can be elusive. If Sir Charles Symonds were writing today about a "particular variety of headache," he would be referring not to cluster headaches, as he was in his landmark 1956 article in *Brain*, but instead to basilar migraine.

Clinical Description
Bickerstaff wrote the first concise description of basilar migraine (BaM) as a variant of migraine with aura. As described, BaM is a series of migraine attacks commencing with symptoms referable to dysfunction in the territory

of the vertebrobasilar arterial circulation. Patients complain of visual disturbances, vertigo, ataxia, dysarthria, tinnitus, and sensory disturbances of distal parts of the limbs and around the lips, followed by throbbing, occipital headache. The International Headache Society (IHS) definition of BaM in its *Classification and Diagnostic Criteria for Headache Disorders, Cranial Neuralgias and Facial Pain* is "migraine with aura originating from the brain stem or both occipital lobes." The headaches must fulfill criteria outlined in the Table.

In his original description, Bickerstaff described 34 adolescent female patients, 80% of whom had a positive family history of migraine headache. In the intervening decades, the perception of basilar migraine as an ailment of female teenagers has remained.

Lapkin and Golden echoed this sentiment but also found the condition to be far more common than previously suspected (23 new cases seen over an 18-month period). Hockaday, while still affirming BaM as a childhood disease, further modified older clinical impressions by demonstrating a male prevalence in her study, the largest to date.

At the Cleveland Clinic, our cases have been culled from an adult referral base of a large Midwestern tertiary-care hospital, and represent an adult headache clinic experience, although a few adolescent patients have been referred. Over a 12-month period, we have seen 47 patients suffering from both BaM and POTS; the median age of the population is 31.5 years, with a range of 18 to 58 years. Four patients were 19 years or younger, and 30% were male. The condition started in the third or fourth decade in more than 80% of the patients, suggesting a clinical experience associated with BaM that extends well outside the boundaries of childhood and adolescence.

The spectra of clinical symptoms are what distinguish BaM from the more routine migraine with aura. Paramount in importance is the bilaterality of the signs and symptoms, related to the anatomic distribution of basilar arterial blood flow.

In the most revealing study to date, Sturzenegger and Meienberg described the clinical picture of 49 patients with definite BaM. While only 57% had occipital headaches, 86% suffered from visual impairment simultaneously involving both visual fields. This was followed by vertigo (63%) and ataxia (63%), bilateral paresthesias (61%), weakness, and dysarthria (both 57%).

Furthermore, disorders of consciousness were seen in 77%, in the form of syncope, confusion, and/or amnesia; 6% were comatose and 8% had seizures. The EEG was abnormal in all patients with altered consciousness, showing predominantly slow wave activity. Interictal EEGs were normal.

For the patients who did not meet extant criteria for BaM (before 1988), the differential diagnosis included epilepsy, vertebral basilar insufficiency, orthostatic hypotension, and hysteria. To this list we would add multiple sclerosis.

Others have commented on epilepsy and the presence of EEG abnormalities in patients with BaM. In a remarkable case, Frequin et al presented a 25-year-old patient with recurrent episodes of reversible coma associated with BaM. Extensive workup showed angiographically documented rostral basilar artery spasm, and EEG monitoring revealed simultaneous frontal intermittent rhythmic delta activity.

Camfield et al documented a series of severe continuous EEG abnormali-

Table. Diagnostic Criteria For Basilar Migraine

- Fulfills criteria for migraine with aura (IHS 1.2)
- Two or more aura symptoms of the following type are present:
- Visual symptoms in both the temporal and nasal fields of both eyes
- Slurred speech or dysarthria
- Vertigo
- Tinnitus
- Decreased hearing
- Double vision
- Ataxia
- Bilateral paresthesias
- Bilateral weakness
- Decreased level of consciousness

ties accompanying BaM—unilateral or bilateral temporo-occipital spike, spike/wave, or spike and slow wave. All abnormalities were reversible and ultimately benign findings. Swanson and Vick reported a BaM in an adult captured as a photoconvulsive episode on EEG. The patient's condition responded to antiepileptic therapy.

An equally intriguing area of BaM study is the connection of migraine with dizziness and vertigo. Vertigo is a symptom recognized by IHS criteria as a manifestation of BaM. Benign paroxysmal (positional) vertigo of childhood is considered a diagnostic category (IHS 1.5.1), but no such category exists for adults.

Cutrer and Baloh have proposed several explanations for the association of dizziness and migraine. Short episodes of dizziness, such as those occuring during aura, may represent a cortical spreading depression similar to non-basilar auras (see chapters by Green and Aurora). There may be a release of neuro-inflammatory peptides, such as calcitonin gene–related peptide, by trigeminal input to the vestibular nuclei, which would in turn sensitize vestibular neurons to other afferent input, resulting in motion sickness, dizziness, or cyclic vomiting.

Our experience resembles that of Moretti and Manzoni. More than 20 years ago, they described 5 cases of "benign recurrent vertigo" associated with migraine; all had normal neurologic and neuro-otologic examinations.

Further characterization of their cases revealed a high prevalence in women, a high recurrence of attacks, a time correlation with menses, and absence of cochlear and neurologic abnormalities. Moreover, they found a significant family history of migraine and no clear correlation between vertigo and migraine headache attack.

Clinically, all their cases closely resemble what we would label basilar migraine–postural tachycardia syndrome (BaM-POTS). The latter designation refers to orthostatic intolerance or autonomic instability (symptomatic orthostatic tachycardia, diastolic or systolic hypotension) not attributable to an otherwise known cause of autonomic failure. Whether the autonomic instability responsible for symptoms is due to a "migrainous" phenomenon such as a brain-stem neuronal depression or to secondary causes, such as ischemia, is unknown. The 2 cases presented above were representative of the BaM-POTS syndrome.

Treatment

There are no studies that address the treatment of these complex migraine cases in a randomized, double-blind, placebo-controlled fashion. Whereas the acute management of migraine with aura has advanced since the advent of the triptan class of medication, product inserts for triptans advise *against* their use in BaM. The existence of basilar migraine, along with hemiplegic migraine, was one of the criteria for exclusion from triptan clinical trials. There remains the overriding concern within the clinical and pharmaceutical communities that the use of vasoconstrictive agents, such as the triptans and the ergots, could transform a prolonged aura into a permanent deficit.

Review of the old literature, however, shows that many patients in the larger series were treated with dihydroergotamine (DHE) or ergonovine (Ergotrate). These drugs were used, both acutely and prophylactically, without ill effect.

In current practice, other therapeutic approaches, such as the use of antiemetics, either alone or in combination with nonsteroidal anti-inflammatory drugs, can be safe and effective. Intravenous valproate (Depakote) can be used in an infusion unit and has shown efficacy anecdotally. Prevention of BaM would be identical to principles described in treating migraine with and without auras (see Finkel, Green, and Aurora chapters). Particularly in this class of headache disorders, where deficits can be both prolonged and disabling, the role of prevention is paramount.

Conclusion

Both cases represent the difficult diagnostic and management issues seen in patients with basilar migraine. Case 1 resembles the typical chronic daily headache more than it does basilar migraine, with some exceptions. As with many chronic headache cases, the patient suffers from psychological comorbidity and had at some point been overusing immediate-relief analgesics. Also, as with other patients with migraine with and without aura, the patient had a positive family history for migraine and a normal workup.

What distinguished this patient, of course, was the history of unusual auras. The symptoms were bilateral and suggested dysfunction of bilateral striate cortices and the rostral brain stem (eg, diplopia and confusion, syncope). While some of the symptoms could last for hours, there was no radiographic evidence, on diffusion MR imaging, of stroke. Nevertheless, potential vasoconstrictors were avoided as abortive agents, despite reports of safe use of DHE and ergonovine in the 1970s and 1980s.

The second patient emphasizes the diagnostic difficulties encountered in these cases. This patient was dismissed as hysterical by an experienced neurologist, and although she had significant psychological comorbidity, her condition was remediable.

As in the first case, there appears to be an association between the aura of BaM and the brain stem's control of autonomic functions such as heart rate and blood pressure. While it remains speculation, the association between symptoms such as bilateral visual distortion, vertigo, hearing loss, tinnitus, bilateral weakness and paresthesias, and brain-stem autonomic function seems apparent.

Moretti and Manzoni described 5 cases of "benign recurrent vertigo" similar to the above-mentioned cases. POTS had not been accepted as a clinical phenomenon yet, but their patients probably would have met diagnostic criteria as outlined by Low et al in the selected reading below.

How can such a profound clinical syndrome as BaM leave no permanent deficits? It seems unlikely that a primary ischemic phenomenon could leave so few traces, and this makes more attractive as an explanation for migraine aura the theory of spreading neuronal depression referred to in the Green (page 58) and Aurora (page 105) chapters. Much more exploratory work needs to be done.

Editors' Note

We can't resist discussing prevention a bit more. As Dr. Stillman noted, prevention is extremely important in these patients, because of the disability associated with their aura and the hesitancy to use the migraine-specific triptans.

As noted in Dr. Landy's chapter (page 116), it is possible that complex, prolonged auras are related to calcium channelopathy caused by mutations in the P/Q type calcium channel α_{1A}-subunit (*CACNA1A*) gene on chromosome 19p13 (Terwindt et al). Because patients with familial hemiplegic migraine respond so well to conventional calcium channel blockers, we at the New England Center for Headache use these medications as our first-line preventive agents in patients with migraine with aura. The more challenging the aura, the more likely we are to use them.

As ß-blockers have been described anecdotally to exacerbate aura in some patients, we eschew them at the beginning, although we have seen many patients with migraine with aura do very well on prophylactic ß-blocker treatment. And because we agree with Dr. Stillman that aura is primarily a neurologic event and not a vascular event, we frequently use antiepileptic drugs for prevention.

A link has been made between cortical spreading depression, channelopathy, and mitochondrial dysfunction. Because of this interrelationship, the use of riboflavin to increase ATP production in the electron transport chain in the mitochondria to correct abnormalities manifesting in phosphorylation defects has been championed by Schoenen. We find that riboflavin (vitamin B_2) 400 mg per day may be a useful adjunct in the treatment of patients with migraine, especially those with migrainous aura.

Magnesium deficiency intracellularly in the cortex has been shown to be present in migraineurs. In patients who can tolerate chelated magnesium 400 to 600 mg per day, additional benefit can sometimes be seen. Thus, it is often our custom to use a calcium channel blocker or antiepileptic drug with riboflavin and magnesium in patients who merit preventive treatment.

Many headache specialists cautiously use triptans in hemiplegic migraine and basilar migraine even though it is prohibited to do so according to the prescribing information for all of the triptans. A discussion on the controversy of using triptans in complicated auras can be found in Dr. Landy's chapter.

<u>Diagnosis:</u> Basilar Migraine and Postural Orthostatic Tachycardia Syndrome

Selected Reading

Bickerstaff ER. Basilar artery migraine. *Lancet.* 1961;1:15-17.

Bickerstaff ER. Impairment of consciousness in migraine. *Lancet* 1961;2:1057-1059.

Camfield PR, Metrakos K, Andermann F. Basilar migraine, seizures, and severe epileptiform EEG abnormalities. *Neurology.* 1978;28:584-588.

Cutrer FM, Baloh RW. Migraine-associated dizziness. *Headache.* 1992;32:300-304.

Ferguson KS, Robinson SS. Life-threatening migraine. *Arch Neurol.* 1982;39:374-376.

Frequin ST, Linssen WH, Pasman JW, et al. Recurrent prolonged coma due to basilar artery migraine: a case report. *Headache.* 1991;31:75-81.

Headache Classification Committee of the Internetaional Headache Society. Classification and Diagnostic Criteria for Headache Disorders, Cranial Neuralgias and Facial Pain. *Cephalalgia.* 1988;8(suppl 7):1-96.

Hockaday JM. Basilar migraine in childhood. *Dev Med Child Neurol.* 1979;21:455-463.

Kayan A, Hood JD. Neuro-otological manifestations of migraine. *Brain.* 1984;107:1123-1142.

Lance JW, Anthony M. Some clinical aspects of migraine. *Arch Neurology.* 1966;15:356-361.

Lapkin ML, Golden GS. Basilar artery migraine. *Am J Dis Child.* 1978;132:278-281.

Low PA, Opfer-Gehrking TL, Textor SC, et al. Postural tachycardia syndrome (POTS). *Neurology.* 1995;45(suppl 5):S19-S25.

Moretti G, Manzoni GC. "Benign recurrent vertigo" and its connection with migraine. *Headache.* 1980;20:344-346.

Neuhauser H, Leopold M, von Brevern M, et al. The interrelations of migraine, vertigo, and migraine vertigo. *Neurology.* 2001;56:436-441.

Schoenen J, Jacquy J, Lenaerts M. Effectiveness of high-dose riboflavin in migraine prophylaxis. A randomized controlled trial. *Neurology.* 1998;50:466-470.

Sturzenegger MH, Meienberg O. Basilar artery migraine: a follow-up study of 82 cases. *Headache.* 1985;25:408-415.

Swanson JW, Vick NA. Basilar artery migraine: 12 patients, with an attack recorded electroencephalographically. *Neurology.* 1978;28:782-786.

Symonds C. A particular variety of headache. *Brain.* 1956;79:217.

Terwindt GM, Ophoff RA, van Eijk R, et al. Dutch Migraine Genetics Research Group. Involvement of the *CACNA1A* gene containing region on 19p13 in migraine with and without aura. *Neurology.* 2001;56:1028-1032.

15. The Man With Persistent Visual Symptoms

Sheena K. Aurora, MD

Co-director, Swedish Headache Center
Swedish Neurosciences Institute
Seattle, Washington

Case

A 39-year-old filmmaker was referred by his neurologist for a second opinion for persistent visual phenomena.

The visual phenomena consisted of small "fuzzy holes." The holes slowly became larger over several minutes, eventually encompassing half of the man's visual field. This was followed by a severe headache associated with nausea and vomiting. The visual symptoms lasted a few hours and resolved before the start of the headache. The headaches partially responded to a butalbital combination, but the subject was always left with a mild headache, similar to a 24-hour hangover. He had headaches approximately once or twice a month, and the usual trigger was stress or the "letdown" following stress. The subject occasionally experienced head pain triggered by light.

The patient noticed with each headache that although his visual symptoms resolved, he was left with faint squiggly lines and a slight haze in his entire visual field. He would usually notice this while looking at the sky or a flat white wall. His headaches were effectively prevented with propranolol or verapamil, and the frequency was reduced to only once or twice a year. However, the haze/visual phenomena were persistent when headaches did occur.

The visual disturbance worsened with every headache. Over the next few years, the visual phenomenon was described as "snowy vision," which was present all the time and would worsen episodically, unassociated with pain. The subject described the visual phenomenon as like looking at a television with bad reception. It moved and swirled, and covered his entire visual field. When he looked at the sky or a white wall, the snowy effect was dark gray. He also saw constant "sparks," "shooting stars," and "floaters." When the patient closed his eyes or looked at a dark surface, he saw the same effects, except that all of the visual phenomena were white, similar to looking at a sky full of moving and shooting stars.

The visual phenomena were least noticeable when the man looked at surfaces or objects that had middle tones mixed with textures, shadows, and colors, or had dull, rough surfaces. The visual phenomena then seemed to blend into objects (eg, a textured wall). The visual phenomena were also less noticeable when he was watching television or movies and most profound when he was looking at flat or shiny, 1-color surfaces.

The patient had tried various medications for the visual phenomena, including antiepileptic drugs such as divalproex sodium (Depakote, oral and intravenous), lamotrigine (Lamictal), gabapentin (Neurontin), carbamazepine, and topiramate (Topamax). Other prophylactic agents utilized were cyproheptadine, methylphenidate, sertraline (Zoloft), acetazolamide, baclofen, coenzyme Q10, magnesium oxide, and feverfew. The only medication that produced an improvement, albeit mild, was baclofen. This was at high doses, however, and also produced sedation, making it difficult for the patient to participate in normal activities.

Family History
Significant for a mother with similar headaches and definite visual aura.

Past Medical History and Review of Systems
Consistent with good health.

General and Neurologic Exams
Normal in all respects.

Discussion
This patient experienced both migraine with aura and migraine aura without headache. The aura associated with migraine is a fascinating phenomenon and has been a puzzle to migraine sufferers, clinicians, and scientists alike. Only 20% of migraineurs experience aura; even then, it is not present with every migraine attack.

Migraine aura without headache, as exemplified by this illustrative case, is a less common phenomenon. It occurs commonly in patients who have had migraine with aura or in relatives of patients with migraine. This case is an extreme example of prolonged or persistent visual aura without migraine headache, and represents one end of the spectrum.

For most patients, the migraine aura without headache is episodic and lasts 15 to 30 minutes. This has been variously called a "migrainous equivalent," "visual migraine," or late-life migraine accompaniment (when it occurs in late middle age or later), and, incorrectly, "retinal migraine" (a unilateral retinal

Table. Selected Antiepileptic Drugs for Migraine

Drug	Efficacy	Side Effects	Relative Contraindication	Relative Indication
Divalproex	4+	2+	Liver disease, bleeding disorders	Mania, epilepsy, impulse control
Topiramate	3+	2+	Kidney stones	Epilepsy, mania, neuropathic pain
Gabapentin	2+	2+		Epilepsy, neuropathic pain

Adapted from: Silberstein SD, et al. Headache for the Primary Care Physician. 2000.
Gray RN, et al. *US Dept of Health and Human Services.* 1999.

artery spasm rather than a cortical event).

The mechanism of migraine with aura has been better elucidated over the past decade with the help of noninvasive technology. Harold G. Wolff, a pioneer of the vascular theory of migraine, proposed that the neurologic symptoms of the migraine aura were caused by cerebral vasoconstriction, and the headache by vasodilatation of the arteries of the scalp.

Lashley's experience of his own visual aura led him to the concept of cortical spreading depression (CSD) of Leão as the primary cause, a discharge precipitated by injury to the visual cortex of laboratory animals. This promulgates a neural rather than a vascular cause for migraine aura.

Abnormal cortical or neuronal excitability has been suggested as a possible factor predisposing to the phenomenon of CSD. The pathophysiologic basis of the migraine aura appears related to firing of excitable nerves in the occipital cortex, which initiates CSD that moves anteriorly over the cortex. This, in turn, produces the aura.

In a rare form of inherited migraine with prolonged hemiplegic aura (familial hemiplegic migraine), the genes for about half of affected families have been cloned and found on chromosome 1 or 19. These mutant genes code for abnormal calcium channels, which may lead to firing of hyperexcitable neurons and result in severe aura. This is further evidence of a neuronal basis for aura.

The unpredictable and elusive nature of migraine has prevented many investigators from systematically studying migraine aura. Recent research by Cao et al, in which migraine was reliably visually triggered in 50% of subjects, enabled immediate measurement of early events of the migraine aura attack. Using newly developed functional magnetic resonance imaging techniques, the investigators were able to show in some patients with aura a slow neuronal change in the occipital cortex, moving forward at a rate of 3 to 6 mm per minute. Contrary to what we would have expected with Wolff's vascular theory, these patients showed vasodilatation and tissue hyperoxygenation at the spreading edge of the aura, suggesting increased neuronal activity. Obviously, the brain was not ischemic during the aura.

Treatment

The treatment for persistent migraine aura is based on the neuronal theory of hyperexcitability, with the mainstay of first-line treatment being antiepileptic drugs. Most patients in my experience (unlike the illustrative case) respond well to low dosages of antiepileptic drugs, There is strong scientific evidence for the use of divalproex sodium (500-1,500 mg/day), gabapentin (1,800-2,700 mg/day), and topiramate (50-150 mg/day) (Table). These medications have demonstrated effective prevention of migraine, with at least 1 double-blind, placebo-controlled study confirming the efficacy of each. There are anecdotal reports for lamotrigine, levetiracetam (Keppra), tiagabine (Gabitril), and zonisamide (Zonegran). These drugs have not been studied in the subpopulation of migraine aura without headache.

However, since there is a unifying neuronal mechanism, there is indirect evidence for a proof of concept.

Calcium channel blockers may also work in the treatment of migraine aura without headache. Familial hemiplegic migraine, as noted above, is caused by mutant voltage-gated P/Q-type calcium channel genes, which likely influence presynaptic neurotransmitter release, possibly of excitatory amino acid systems. Currently, there are no drugs designed as blockers for the P/Q calcium channel. Verapamil, which is a peripheral calcium channel blocker, is effective for patients with migraine with aura who have basilar type symptoms; it has also been found to be very effective in familial hemiplegic migraine at doses of 240-480 mg per day. Acetazolamide, a carbonic anhydrase inhibitor, may work at doses of 500-1,000 mg per day.

Using nuclear magnetic resonance spectroscopy, Ramadan et al demonstrated low intracellular magnesium in the occipital cortex of patients with familial hemiplegic migraine. Therefore, chelated magnesium supplementation, at doses of 400-600 mg per day, may also be effective in some patients.

Finally, Schoenen found vitamin B_2 or riboflavin particularly useful in patients with aura, at a dose of 400 mg per day maintained for at least 3 to 4 months. This may be due to flavinoids correcting a mitochondrial problem in energy production in the electron transport chain in aura, which may also lead to neuronal firing.

As there have been no medications shown effective in double-blind, placebo-controlled studies in migraine aura without headache, the selection of treatment is necessarily empiric and anecdotal. Most patients elect no treatment if the disorder is episodic. For persistent visual aura, the antiepileptics work best in my experience. Noninvasive investigation—ie, functional magnetic resonance imaging and magnetoencephalography—will allow us to further elucidate causative mechanisms and, from there, to develop targeted treatment.

Editors' Note

Dr. Aurora presents an excellent example of migraine with aura and aura without migraine pain. Given the fact that the 2 can occur in the same patient, as can migraine without aura, some investigators have suggested that migraine and aura may indeed be separate phenomena, existing on parallel pathophysiologic tracks in which the process of aura may induce the headache phase in biologically susceptible individuals and not in others. On the opposing side are those who believe aura is always present but may occur in "silent" areas of the brain. Triptans are approved and effective in migraine with aura and migraine without aura. They have not been found to be helpful in shortening aura.

We do permit oral dosing of triptans during typical aura, and in some lucky patients this appears to prevent or truncate the migraine that follows, although no prospective studies confirm this.

Diagnosis: Migraine Aura Without Headache, Migraine With Aura

Selected Reading

Bowyer SM, Aurora SK, Moran JE, et al. Magnetoencephalographic fields from patients with spontaneous and induced migraine aura. *Ann Neurol.* 2001;50:582-587.

Cao Y, Welch KMA, Aurora SK, Vikingstad EM. Functional MRI-BOLD of visually triggered headache and visual change in migraine sufferers. *Arch Neurol.* 1999;56:548-554.

. The Woman With Monthly Headaches

Merle Diamond, MD, FACEP

Medical Director, Diamond Headache Inpatient Unit
Associate Director, Diamond Headache Clinic
Clinical Assistant Professor, Department of Medicine,
Finch University Health Sciences/Chicago Medical School
Chicago, Illinois

5-year-old professor at a local college, was referred with a 30-year
f migraine without aura.

tient experienced 4 attacks per month. She had 2 or 3 attacks
d throughout the month and then a single prolonged attack asso-
th her menstrual cycle. She used sumatriptan (Imitrex) 100 mg
sumatriptan 6 mg subcutaneously for the sporadic monthly
vith excellent response. KS usually required one dose of medica-
was pain-free within a short time. When treated early, her
s were usually not disabling, and she did not complain of head-
rrence.

nately, KS experienced a more prolonged and difficult-to-manage
associated with her menstrual cycle. These headaches would typi-
r during the late luteal phase and continue for 4 to 5 days. Occa-
ese migraine attacks lasted up to 14 days.

at times been completely disabled by the attacks. In the past 2
has gone to the emergency department to be "knocked out"—her
tive medications can take the "edge" off the pain but do not allow
tion—approximately 4 times.

patient has experienced early menopause, her periods have
ore irregular, and she feels that her headaches are becoming
y difficult to manage. She has also complained of difficulty falling
g asleep, as well as occasional autonomic symptoms of warmth
resis. She wonders if her headaches would resolve if she under-
terectomy.

al History and Review of Systems

diagnosed with hyperlipidemia. The patient does not drink or

ory

or a father with late-life coronary artery disease and hypertension,
er with migraine.

nd Laboratory Workup

Lashley KS. Patterns of cerebral integration indicated by th[
Neurol Psychol. 1941;46:331-339.

Leão AAP. Spreading depression of activity in the cerebral [
8:379-390.

Ramadan NM, Halverson H, Vande-Linde A, et al. Low bra[
Headache. 1989;29:416-419.

Schoenen J, Jacquy J, Lenaerts M. Effectiveness of high-[
phylaxis. A randomized controlled trial. *Neurology.* 1998;5[

Welch KM, D'Andrea G, Tepley N, Barkley G, Ramadan N[
state of central neuronal hyperexcitability. *Neurol Clin.* 19[

Case
   KS, a [
history [

   The p[
scattere[
ciated [
orally o[
attacks,[
tion and[
migraine[
ache rec[

   Unfort[
migraine[
cally occ[
sionally, t[

   KS has[
years, she[
usual abo[
her to fu[

   As the[
become [
increasing[
and stayi[
and diaph[
went a hy[

Past Medi[
   Recently[
smoke.

Family His[
   Positive [
and a moth[

Diagnostic[
   Normal.

General and Neurologic Exam
Normal.

Discussion
Migraine preferentially affects women once they reach adulthood. Many women complain that their migraine attacks are more frequent and difficult to manage during menses and the perimenopausal period.

The prevalence of menstrual migraine is an area of some controversy. It is not recognized as a separate entity by the International Headache Society (IHS). As noted in Dr. Newman's chapter, 70% of women have menstrually associated headaches, but cases of true menstrual migraine (whereby women experience migraine only with their menstrual cycle) are much more rare, occurring in about 7% or 8% of patients. A large diary study by Stewart and Lipton reported that patients complaining of menstrual migraine had more frequent attacks around the time of their menstrual cycle. The duration and severity of these attacks were not significantly different from those of their other migraine attacks.

This study was perhaps not reflective of patients seen in our office, as patients who consult us or other specialists may have higher levels of headache-related disability. In other words, the study patients may not have consulted a healthcare professional for migraine management.

The most important issue is that this patient is likely perimenopausal, and migraine increases in frequency and severity during this stage of life, as evidenced by data from epidemiologic studies. Particular factors that may emerge include comorbidites such as depression, anxiety, vasomotor instability, and sleep disorders. This patient presents with many issues that must be addressed in the aging migraine population, such as the addition of risk factors for vascular disease.

Treatment
First, we must address the patient's chief complaint: menstrual migraine in a perimenopausal period, with irregular periods and significant headaches. In any patient consulting for menstrual migraine, a thorough history is important. Maintaining a headache calendar can be very helpful in planning an appropriate therapy.

Most patients use migraine-specific drugs (triptans)—which can work effectively during their menstrual cycle—on an as-needed basis, even if the periods become irregular. There have been numerous studies of acute treatment of menstrual migraine with triptans. These studies have demonstrated that triptans are equally efficacious during the menstrual migraine and the nonmenstrual attack.

Some patients may benefit from longer treatment periods during the menstrual cycle, but will respond well to standard therapy. As Dr. Newman noted, the second option is to use focal management, or what is often called "miniprophylaxis." This involves using nonsteroidal anti-inflammatory drugs or triptans daily, beginning several days before the expected onset of the menstrual migraine. However, the problem for this patient and those like her is that her periods are now irregular and no longer predictable.

Options for treating menstrual headaches also include adding an anti-dopaminergic agent such as chlorpromazine or metoclopramide. These agents can act as abortive drugs in migraine. Some of these agents, however, can cause sedation or extrapyramidal symptoms.

For prolonged headaches, a short course of corticosteroids can be used, such as dexamethasone tablets or a methylprednisolone dose pack. This therapy should not be used more often than once a month. If this form of treatment is needed frequently, supplementation with calcium and vitamin D may be suggested to prevent osteoporosis.

Migraines associated with the menstrual cycle are thought to be related to hormonal fluctuations, especially decreases in estrogen production associated with the late luteal phase. Therefore, supplementation with an estrogen patch has been suggested. Unfortunately, owing to normal variations of a woman's cycle, this treatment is often difficult to time appropriately; this was particularly true in this perimenopausal woman.

If the patient experiences regular menses, initiation of treatment with a low-strength estradiol patch can be helpful, starting around cycle day 21 or 22. If the lowest strength is not helpful, it may be appropriate to increase the dose of the patch. Trials for menstrual migraine treatment should be done over 3 to 4 cycles to determine success or failure. In women using continuous oral contraceptive packs, limiting the number of menstrual migraine attacks by limiting the frequency of menstrual cycles can be helpful.

Historically, oral contraceptives have been avoided in migraine patients because of the likelihood of increasing the frequency and severity of attacks. Older preparations with high doses of estrogen often provoked more significant migraine attacks. Newer, lower-dose estrogen–progesterone compounds are often well tolerated.

Because of this patient's strong family history of coronary artery disease and stroke, and the recent onset of hyperlipidemia, oral contraceptives early in the perimenopausal period might not be appropriate.

For any patient with migraine desiring to use oral contraceptives, education regarding risk/benefit should be done. It is also important to limit risk factors in these patients. Patients should maintain a headache diary to ascertain that their headache frequency is not exacerbated by oral contraceptives. In women who tolerate oral contraceptive consecutive pill packs for 3 to 4 months, the process of planned menses can be beneficial.

Several other approaches to the treatment of menstrual migraine have been studied. Daily dihydroergotamine by injection or nasal spray can be used during the days of headache. Usually, an antiemetic is added to this protocol. The use of methysergide during at-risk days is another intervention.

Some physicians advocate the use of preventive drugs for brief periods during the menstrual cycle, although there are limited data to support this concept. Finally, a logical approach in patients who are refractory to most therapies is to use standard preventive therapy daily.

In selection of a preventive agent, it is important to consider comorbidities. For example, in this patient and others who are perimenopausal, hyperlipidemia and increasing vascular risk factors may indicate a need to avoid β-blockers, which can increase lipid values.

Many perimenopausal women have comorbid depression or anxiety. The use of a tricyclic antidepressant in a small dose may help with sleep disturbances and migraine frequency. It is very important to discuss preventive treatment outcomes, duration of therapy, goals for decreasing headache frequency and severity, and potential for side effects.

For example, some medications used for prevention increase a patient's appetite. This is particularly true of the older sedative tricyclics, as well as divalproex sodium (Depakote) and some other antiepileptic drugs. Since many women are prone to weight gain (approximately 10 pounds) while going through menopause, it is important to warn them regarding the possibility of food cravings. Education may be needed to increase patient compliance and diminish side effects.

Because of the level of disability and duration of this woman's menstrual migraines, it is likely that she will have a better outcome with standard prevention. This favorable prognosis needs to be discussed with the patient.

Another nonpharmacologic approach to menstrual migraine is good personal "health hygiene," including regular sleep habits, regular meals, and exercise. Patients who are proactive in their health maintenance seem to do better. There are data that show regular exercise can decrease both tension-type and migraine headaches. Other data demonstrate that supplementation of 500 mg of elemental magnesium may be helpful in menstrual migraine. This benign intervention can be helpful in our patients.

As with many other perimenopausal women, this patient asked whether surgical menopause might be the answer. Since her worst headaches occur during her menses, why not just get rid of the entire system? Unfortunately, the data on surgical menopause and migraine outcome are not particularly positive.

A study by Neri et al demonstrated that the aging ovary may somehow be protective with respect to migraine frequency. In Neri's series of patients, 70% of subjects who underwent a natural menopause had a reduction in their headaches, compared with 30% of subjects who underwent surgical menopause. Most disturbingly, the condition of 60% of surgical menopause patients actually worsened.

There are other issues that need to be addressed in this patient. The first involves triptan use as she approaches and completes menopause. The second issue is potential hormone replacement therapy in the migraine patient. Over a lifetime, a migraine patient may need to adjust therapies according to the requirements of concomitant medical problems or conditions. Gender-specific problems include pregnancy, breast feeding, and menopause.

Triptans have been available in the United States since 1993. For the vast majority of patients with disabling migraine attacks, these migraine-specific medications provide significant relief. However, triptans are contraindicated in patients with coronary artery disease. Unfortunately, postmenopausal women were often excluded from the triptan clinical trials. Some women continue to be excluded from the use of these drugs simply because they are postmenopausal.

It is important that all patients are assessed for coronary risk factors and individual decisions are made whether that patient is a good candidate for vasoactive medications. Age alone should not warrant exclusion, but it is important to assess each patient's cumulative risks when one is trying to decide appropriate therapy.

In this patient, the only risk factor is hyperlipidemia. Her father suffered from coronary artery disease later in life. This history would not generally be considered a risk factor, as it was not premature vascular disease. To help assess appropriate migraine medication use, it is important to discuss risk factors with patients as they age.

It was very likely that triptan use would have been safe for this patient at this time in her life. The Framingham Study is a good resource for assessment of the appropriateness of a particular therapy in relation to coronary risk factors.

In peri- or postmenopausal patients with excessive cardiovascular risk factors, the use of nonsteroidal anti-inflammatory drugs in combination with metoclopramide may be helpful. If the headaches are frequent and disabling, standard prophylaxis may be needed.

The last issue that should be addressed is the use of hormone replacement therapy (HRT) in the migraine patient. Historically, as with the use of oral contraceptives, many patients were warned regarding the risk of exacerbating migraine with the use of these agents. Certainly, the older treatments containing cyclic estrogens and progestin-induced menses were not particularly helpful and often predictably increased migraine frequency and severity.

During the past decade, HRT has become a much more popular therapy because of possible links to decreasing risks of coronary artery disease, osteoporosis, and dementia. Recently, these ideas were turned on their head, with prospective data from a federally sponsored study finding increased vascular risks with estrogen–progesterone replacement therapy and no evidence of efficacy in preventing dementia, although favorable results for osteoporosis.

During menopause, many women experience autonomic dysfunction, osteoporosis, depression, decreased libido, and sleep disturbances. In menopause, continuous estrogen replacement with progesterone has become a conventional treatment, now quickly being abandoned.

The benefits for the heart must be considered controversial at best, and must be coupled with issues regarding risk factors for breast cancer. Ultimately, with the information we currently have, whether to use HRT is often an individual decision the patient will make, based on autonomic dysfunction, risk of osteoporosis, and family history, especially for vascular disease. The decision whether to use HRT should not be based on the presence of migraine, as the result of HRT on migraine cannot be easily predicted.

If the patient does decide to undergo HRT, a discussion of risk/benefit should occur. Because the effect of HRT on migraine is unpredictable, it is advisable to monitor the headache diary for headache frequency and severity. Some data suggest that estradiol products, particularly patches, may be somewhat better tolerated than conjugated estrogen tablets.

Normally, use of the lowest dose to alleviate the autonomic symptoms is best for the migraine patient. If the patient has an intact uterus, progesterone should be added to the treatment protocol in some way to prevent uterine neoplasm.

Many patients use homeopathic and/or natural remedies. At the time of this writing, about one third of female migraineurs have used traditional HRT (although this number is dropping), while closer to 50% are using other remedies. It is important to determine which products the patient is using in order to limit drug–drug interactions and monitor clinical progress.

Editors' Note

The patient who is perimenopausal presents several clinical challenges. First, there is often a worsening of migraine in premenopause, with improvement after menopause. Second, the issue of HRT often complicates the evaluation of treatment, with respect to efficacy and side effects. Third, the accumulation of vascular risk factors (not gender-specific) requires re-evaluation with respect to vasoactive migraine-specific therapy (triptans). The recent Women's Health Initiative study, as noted by Dr. Diamond, has brought into question some of the benefits of estrogen–progesterone therapy and suggests that there is a slight chance of increased risk of certain conditions such as heart disease, breast cancer, and stroke with replacement.

With respect to the use of steroids as rescue therapy for perimenopausal patients, it might be useful to consider baseline bone density if steroids are to be used on a more frequent basis, and occasionally monitor this parameter. If the patient already has a bone density problem, steroids should be used rarely and under careful supervision, if at all. Dr. Diamond describes beautifully the many factors to be considered and approaches to be taken in the peri- and postmenopausal patient.

<u>Diagnosis:</u> Perimenopausal Migraine

Selected Reading

MacGregor EA. Menstrual migraine: towards a definition. *Cephalalgia*. 1996;16:11-21.

Nappi RE, Cagnacci A, Granella F, et al. Course of primary headaches during hormone replacement therapy. *Maturitas*. 2001;38:157-163.

Neri I, Granolla F, Nappi R, et al. Characteristics of headache at menopause: a clinico-epidemiological study. *Maturitas*. 1993;17:31-37.

Stewart WF, Lipton RB, Chee E, Sawyer J, Silberstein SD. Menstrual cycle and headache. *Neurology*. 2000;55:1517-1523.

Tepper SJ. Safety and rational use of the triptans. *Med Clin North Am*. 2001;85:959-971.

Wernke SM, Martin VT, Zoma WD, et al. The role of gonadotropin-releasing hormone (GnRH) agonists with oestrogen add-back therapy in migraine prevention [abstract]. *Cephalalgia*. 2002;21:449-450.

Writing Group for the Women's Health Initiative Investigators. Risks and benefits of estrogen plus progestin in healthy postmenopausal women. *JAMA*. 2002;288:321-333.

17. The Man With Headache And Weakness

Stephen Landy, MD

Associate Clinical Professor of Neurology
University of Tennessee Medical School
Director, Wesley Headache Clinic
Memphis, Tennessee

Case

Mr. C was a healthy 32-year-old, nonsmoking, right-handed male accountant with a 15-year history of headache with left-sided weakness. He initially had episodic headaches of extended duration; in one instance, an episode lasted for 3 days and was accompanied by profound weakness.

At first his headaches were not associated with weakness, and usually involved left unilateral throbbing head pain that, untreated, increased from mild to moderate over 1 to 2 hours. The headaches were associated with nausea, occasional vomiting, photophobia, and phonophobia—all lasting 12 to 24 hours. After administration of 100 mg sumatriptan (Imitrex) at the onset of the mild headache phase, Mr. C typically experienced relief of headache pain and associated symptoms in 1 to 2 hours.

Before implementation of effective prophylactic treatment, Mr. C's headache frequency was between 4 and 6 attacks monthly. With the use of 5 mg of amlodipine (Lotrel) daily and migraine trigger avoidance, frequency was reduced to 1 or 2 attacks monthly. Migraine triggers included monosodium glutamate, red wine, missed meals, minor head trauma, and stress.

Gradually, visual symptoms began to precede the headache attacks; currently, at least 75% of Mr. C's migraine headaches are preceded by a typical aura. The headaches generally consist of a gradual onset over 10 to 30 minutes of right hemiparesis and numbness, and receptive and expressive aphasia lasting 60 to 90 minutes.

Family History

Positive for a grandmother, father, and sister with hemiplegia associated with headaches.

General and Neurologic Exams

Normal during intervals of headache freedom.

Diagnostic Evaluations

Brain magnetic resonance imaging, brain and neck magnetic resonance angiography, electroencephalogram, electrocardiogram, echocardiogram, erythrocyte sedimentation rate, antinuclear antibody, and anticardiolipin antibody all normal or negative.

Discussion

Hemiplegic migraine is a form of migraine characterized by motor weakness during the aura phase. Although the prevalence of hemiplegia before migraine pain is not known with certainty, it is one of the most unusual aura features. Patients often confuse numbness and weakness, and thus the patient's report of weakness may not be reliable, especially in milder cases.

Of more than 1,000 migraineurs who served as the basis for his book *Migraines*, Oliver Sacks found only 2 patients with this symptom. The American Migraine Study II did not even include this symptom in its questionnaire to establish the prevalence of migraine in the general population. However, in its familial form, hemiplegic migraine has greater significance than its low frequency of occurrence would suggest, as it is the first migraine-associated symptom for which a specific genetic lesion has been identified.

Mr. C's age at onset was 17, compared to the typical onset between 10 and 15 years with familial hemiplegic migraine. In general, the age at onset of hemiplegic migraine is earlier than that of migraine without aura, with cases seen in patients as young as 2 years. Initial onset has also been noted in a 75-year-old patient.

The frequency of hemiplegic episodes varies greatly from patient to patient. The typical frequency is reported to be 3 or 4 per year, although some patients experience only a few episodes in a lifetime, while others may experience almost daily attacks.

It is somewhat unusual that Mr. C continues to experience hemiplegic episodes as frequently as he does as an adult. The frequency of attacks often decreases as patients get older, with hemiplegic episodes becoming less frequent after 20 to 25 years of age and possibly ceasing altogether. However, other migraine manifestations may continue despite the cessation of hemiplegic episodes.

In patients with hemiplegic aura, there are few hard-and-fast rules regarding other associated features of migraine episodes, except perhaps that hemiplegia has never been seen as a single, isolated component of the aura. As in Mr. C's case, hemiplegia is always accompanied by paresthesias and often by speech disturbances. In case series, visual auras are commonly reported.

Symptoms typical of basilar migraine are also commonly associated with hemiplegic aura; vertebrobasilar symptoms or signs such as vertigo, diplopia, drop attacks, tinnitus, and gait problems may occur. In some cases, hemiplegia has been accompanied by states of altered or complete loss of consciousness.

Although Mr. C's attacks almost always evolve into headache, this is not universally the case. In approximately 1 in 10 patients, hemiplegia can occur in the absence of headache. Conversely, patients who experience hemiplegic episodes may not experience them with every migraine headache.

Hemiplegic migraine headaches do not differ from conventional migraine in terms of location, quality, severity, or duration. Associated autonomic symptoms are similar to those seen with other forms of migraine (nausea, vomiting, photophobia, and phonophobia). Although weakness is often contralateral to the headache, no consistent relationship between the location of the headache and the side on which the patient experiences weakness has been noticed.

The duration and severity of motor weakness are highly variable, both between patients and within a single patient over time. Arm and leg weakness is most common. The progression of the weakness is slow, with a spreading or marching quality. Weakness may alternate sides or always involve the same side; bilateral symptoms occur in approximately 1 in 4 patients.

Mr. C's weakness typically lasts no more than 90 minutes and, while inconvenient, is hardly debilitating. The majority of hemiplegic episodes last less than 1 hour, but approximately 15% of episodes may last from 1 day to 1 week. Weakness can range from mild to complete paralysis. It appears that longer-lasting attacks are associated with more severe symptoms. Fortunately, more severe episodes occur less frequently.

Like Mr. C, a large portion of patients (as many as 40%) will experience attacks of unusual duration and severity sometime during their lifetime. Atypical attacks will usually occur before the age of 20 and include a prolonged aura lasting several days. They may include impaired consciousness, ranging from confusion to coma, with respiratory failure. Fever or meningismus may also occur.

In some cases, a severe episode is the first hemiplegic episode experienced by a patient. Patients and their families can be reassured that the symptoms usually resolve completely, and there are rarely any residual neurologic deficits evident between hemiplegic episodes.

A majority of patients can identify triggering factors. The 2 most common are stress and minor head trauma. Common triggers of other forms of migraines are typically not involved in hemiplegic migraine, making Mr. C somewhat unusual in this regard. In some cases, hemiplegic symptoms have been provoked by the injection of contrast enhancement media during cerebral angiography. Extreme physical exertion has also been identified as a trigger.

Mr. C's case is notable because of the 3 relatives with similar migraine symptoms. The International Headache Society (IHS) classifies hemiplegic migraine as a form of migraine with aura. If at least one first-degree relative has identical attacks and is similarly affected, the migraine is subgrouped as familial hemiplegic migraine (FHM). A first-degree relative shares 50% of the patient's genes (ie, parent, full sibling, offspring).

Cases of hemiplegic migraine without a family history are often referred to in the literature as "sporadic." Sporadic cases constitute more than 90% of cases of hemiplegic migraine.

FHM is an autosomal dominant condition, meaning that the gene(s) involved is not found on a sex chromosome, and that heterozygotes with the underlying disease gene display the trait. This has important implications.

First, unlike other presentations of migraine that affect women 3 times more frequently, FHM equally affects men and women. Since it is a dominant condition, about 50% of first-degree relatives would be expected to also show this pattern of migraine. However, penetrance of the trait is incomplete, so not every person carrying the gene will experience the symptoms. Also, the status of first-degree relatives may not be known. This can complicate the diagnosis of FHM, and the clinician may need information on more distant relatives to substantiate the diagnosis.

FHM has been linked to 3 different genetic loci. A gene on chromosome

19 has been identified in about 50% to 60% of families. The gene codes for the alpha 1A subunit of a P/Q-type voltage-dependent calcium channel (CACNA1A). When the variant gene is introduced into frog oocytes, it results in abnormally slow closing of the calcium channel. The term "channel-opathies" has been coined to describe diseases resulting from improperly functioning ion channels such as the FHM calcium channels.

In about 20% of families, the trait is linked to chromosome 1, but the relevant gene has yet to be identified. Finally, another 20% of families are not linked to either chromosome 19 or 1, indicating the existence of at least one additional locus. At least one case has been related to a de novo mutation (ie, not inherited) at the CACNA1A site on chromosome 19.

In general, the presentation of FHM does not seem to be influenced by which genetic locus is involved. The severity, frequency, and associated symptoms do not markedly differ by genetic subtype.

In one series, however, it did appear that penetrance was lower in families in which the gene on chromosome 1 was involved. Of greater importance, permanent cerebellar signs have been seen only in families with involvement of the gene on chromosome 19.

Typical of most patients with hemiplegic aura, Mr. C has no residual signs or symptoms between attacks. However, patients with FHM should be examined closely for cerebellar signs, particularly nystagmus and ataxia.

As noted above, these posterior fossa signs are found in some FHM families linked to chromosome 19. Nystagmus is found in about 75% of the family members experiencing hemiplegia, and ataxia in about 40%. Nystagmus is often the first symptom, with progressive ataxia developing later in life. Cerebellar atrophy has been noted in magnetic resonance images of patients with these signs. Other neurologic symptoms have been reported in hemiplegic migraine families, including essential tremor, retinitis pigmentosa, deafness, and cognitive impairment.

Neurologic investigations reveal few remarkable findings during hemiplegic attacks. During severe attacks, some patients will have cerebrospinal fluid (CSF) pleocytosis.

Electroencephalogram (EEG) tracings are abnormal, showing diffuse slow-wave activity predominantly contralateral to the weakness. The EEG changes may persist weeks after the attack. Computed tomography and magnetic resonance images obtained either during or directly after an attack are typically normal except for rare findings of cerebellar atrophy (see above), focal abnormalities of uncertain etiology, and in at least one case, edema of one cerebral hemisphere. Cerebral angiography is typically normal, but there are case reports of arterial constriction and spasm. Since angiography can aggravate the attack, it should be avoided in these patients.

In patients presenting with transient hemiplegia, a thorough workup is necessary to rule out other diagnoses. Other causes of reversible hemiplegia are focal seizures, homocysteinuria, cerebral emboli, carotid and vertebrobasilar dissection, cardiac arrhythmia, meningitis, encephalitis, hypoglycemia, blood chemistry imbalances, organ failure, drug intoxication, and coagulation and connective tissue disorders.

Several uncommon diagnoses are also possible: ornithine transcarbamylase deficiency; mitochondrial myopathy with encephalopathy, lactic acidosis, and stroke-like episodes (MELAS); cerebral autosomal dominant arteriopathy with subcortical infarcts and leukoencephalopathy (CADASIL); and headache with neurologic deficits and CSF lymphocytosis (also referred to as pseudo-migraine with temporary neurologic symptoms and lymphocytic pleocytosis). In Mr. C's case, clinical presentation, normal tests, and brain imaging ruled out most other diagnoses.

Treatment

Mr. C has responded well to nonpharmacologic (trigger avoidance), abortive, and prophylactic migraine treatments. When thinking about treating hemiplegic migraine, one must distinguish between interventions targeting the headache and those targeting the hemiplegic aura. As with any form of migraine, the first step is to avoid identifiable triggers.

The initiation of prophylaxis needs to be considered in light of the complete spectrum of the patient's experience. According to Ducros and Campbell, "In most patients, the hemiplegic attacks are so infrequent that prophylactic therapy is not considered solely to prevent those rare [hemiplegic migraine] episodes."

In Mr. C's case, his attacks were so frequent that he was eager to initiate prophylactic therapy. Because FHM is so uncommon, there are few studies or case series that can serve as a guide; because it is believed to be related to the unusually slow closing of P/Q-type calcium channels, there is some basis to believe that calcium channel blockers may be of benefit. Mr. C was treated with amlodipine, and there are reports in the literature suggesting benefit from flunarizine, verapamil, and nimodipine (Nimotop). Nifedipine can cause headache in many migraineurs and generally should be avoided.

Anticonvulsants have also shown efficacy. Acetazolamide may be of particular benefit in the patients with cerebellar manifestations, as it is used successfully in the hereditary cerebellar ataxias, which are also calcium channelopathies. The use of β-blockers is controversial, but given the evidence that these drugs might be harmful to hemiplegic migraine patients, if used at all, they should be used under careful supervision.

Headache, and not hemiplegia, is the usual focus of abortive therapy in hemiplegic migraine patients. The question is: Is there any reason to treat migraineurs with hemiplegia differently from other migraine patients? Based on the theory that neurologic symptoms are due to the vasoconstriction of intracranial vessels, many physicians avoid prescribing drugs with vasoconstrictive properties. For this reason, triptans and dihydroergotamine have traditionally been avoided, and hemiplegic migraine is currently listed in the prescribing information as a contraindication for use of triptans and ergots.

Several neurologists have published their anecdotal and effective experience with triptans and ergots in treating hemiplegic and basilar migraine, but no prospective, properly powered statistical safety studies have yet been performed. In Mr. C's case, sumatriptan effectively and consistently aborted his headaches. At his request, despite the contraindication, he was given sumatriptan for his migraines after hemiplegic aura, and it has never complicated his hemiparesis. Because of the contraindication and controversy, this approach should never be undertaken without informed consent from the patient, consideration of risks and benefits, and attempts to first treat with preventive medication and nonvasoactive medication.

Abortive therapy in patients experiencing prolonged or severe hemiparesis should certainly be considered. Intravenous verapamil, sublingual nifedipine, and intranasal ketamine have shown benefit in anecdotal reports.

Conclusion

Hemiplegia is a relatively uncommon aura component. It can be frightening, but it is usually benign and self-limited.

Because of the large number of close relatives with similar migraines, Mr. C was diagnosed as having familial hemiplegic migraine. This rare form of migraine is important because it has led to the identification of specific mutations associated with the symptoms. The mutations that have been characterized thus far involve a subunit of the P/Q-type voltage-dependent calcium channel. Whereas discovery of one FHM gene is an important clue for the development of new migraine treatments, the generalizability of the findings in FHM to more common migraine subtypes remains to be established.

These genetic findings presage an era when it may be possible to subtype disease by an underlying genetic basis and allow for treatment that targets the associated physiologic deficit. Until that time, physicians must make use of the best current evidence in managing hemiplegic migraine patients. In most cases, targeting the headache and not the hemiplegia will provide the patient's best chance for an improved quality of life.

Editors' Note

At the New England Center for Headache, we do not usually use triptans and never use ergots in the treatment of hemiplegic or basilar migraine. The anecdotal reports of their effectiveness are not sufficient to reassure us of the safety of this approach. On rare occasions, when a patient comes to us with a personal history of safe and effective use of a triptan with this condition, we have considered continuing careful use of triptans after obtaining informed consent.

Nonetheless, it is very important to remember that the prohibition on triptan and ergot use in these patients stems not from reported adverse events but, rather, from theoretical concerns resulting in the exclusion of these patients from the pivotal studies on triptans and ergots. Triptans have not been shown to be unsafe in this condition; there are just not any adequate data.

Many headache specialists regard hemiplegia as an aura analogous to a visual aura, which is probably neuronal, not vascular. For this reason, some physicians have prescribed triptans in patients with severe symptoms.

Because hemiplegic and basilar migraines are rare, collecting enough patients to establish safety will be very difficult. Thus, the sad state of not knowing whether we are depriving these patients of optimal therapy or whether we are doing them a favor by avoiding potentially harmful medications is likely to persist.

Dr. Lander makes an extremely important point when he comments that patients often confuse weakness (which would contraindicate triptans) and numbness (which would not). Be sure to spend time establishing this distinction with patients before refusing them migraine-specific treatment. Also, reflect on whether the difference between the 2 symptoms should really matter when it comes to a decision to use triptans or not.

Finally, as calcium channel blockers seem to help and β-blockers have been described as worsening this syndrome, we would suggest using effective doses of calcium channel blockers and avoiding the use of β-blockers.

<u>Diagnosis:</u> Familial Hemiplegic Migraine

Selected Reading

Silberstein SD, Lipton RB, Dalessio DJ, eds. *Wolff's Headache and Other Head Pain.* 7th ed. New York, NY: Oxford University Press; 2001.

Ducros A, Campbell JK. Familial hemiplegic migraine. In: Olesen J, Tfelt-Hansen P, Welch KMA, eds. *The Headaches.* 2nd ed. Philadelphia, Pa: Lippincott Williams & Wilkins; 2000.

Ducros A, Joutel A, Vahedi K, et al. Mapping of a second locus for familial hemiplegic migraine to 1q21-23 and evidence of further genetic heterogeneity. *Ann Neurol.* 1997; 42:885-890.

Gardner K. The genetic link to migraine pathophysiology. In: Ramadan N, ed. *Seminars in Headache Management.* Migraine Pathophysiology—Part I. 1999;4(1):2-10.

Gardner K, Barmada MM, Ptacek LJ, et al. A new locus for hemiplegic migraine maps to chromosome 1q31. *Neurology.* 1997;49:1231-1238.

Hans M, Luvisetto S, Williams ME, et al. Functional consequences of mutations in the human alpha1$_A$ calcium channel subunit linked to familial hemiplegic migraine. *J Neurosci.* 1999;19:1610-1619.

Ophoff RA, Terwindt GM, Vergouwe MN, et al. Familial hemiplegic migraine and episodic ataxia type-2 are caused by mutations in the Ca2+ channel gene CACNL1A4. *Cell.* 1996; 87:543-552.

18. The Adolescent Girl With Headaches

Eric M. Pearlman, MD, PhD

Assistant Professor
Mercer University School of Medicine
Georgia Neurological Institute
Savannah, Georgia

Case

MJ, a 14-year-old girl, presented with headaches that had started when she was 6 years of age.

When she was younger, she would stop playing, cry, occasionally vomit, lie down, and go to sleep for 1 to 2 hours. Within the past year, the headaches have increased in frequency, occurring 4 to 6 times per month. MJ noticed that since the start of menstruation, she usually has had 1 or 2 headaches just before the onset of menses.

MJ describes her present headache as throbbing pain across her forehead and behind her eyes. Sometimes it may be more severe behind one eye. She has sensitivity to light and cannot tolerate kitchen or food odors when she has a headache. The headaches are often associated with nausea and occasionally with vomiting. Untreated, they last 6 to 24 hours and are usually relieved with sleep. She has no aura except for some bright "sparkles or stars" associated with her headaches.

MJ has tried acetaminophen and ibuprofen, with limited success. The medications do not completely relieve her pain unless she goes to sleep. Her primary care physician has given her acetaminophen with codeine, which helps her sleep. She has been to the emergency room 3 times in the past year for headaches and, while there, received intravenous pain medication.

MJ has noticed that certain odors, such as that of the cleaning solutions at school, may trigger her headache. She has not noticed any dietary triggers, and has no significant stress at home or school. She avoids slumber parties because she usually gets a headache when she attends one. MJ is an honor student, plays soccer and softball, takes violin lessons, and is active in the Girl Scouts.

MJ suffers from fairly significant motion sickness. Her mother recalls episodes where, as a toddler, MJ would suddenly grab onto her leg, cry, and refuse to walk for about 20 minutes; then she would be fine.

Past Medical History

No other significant medical history.

Family History

About once a month, MJ's mother suffers from "sinus headaches," which are often accompanied by vomiting; she frequently is confined to bed when she has these headaches. MJ's paternal aunt also has migraine.

Diagnostic Workup
Two computed tomography scans yielded normal results.

Exam
General and neurologic exams produced normal results.

Diagnosis and Treatment
MJ was given the diagnosis of migraine without aura. She and her mother were educated on trigger avoidance as well as the benefits of regular sleep, meals, and exercise. She was given a headache diary and instructed on how to complete it, the importance of keeping an accurate diary, and the importance of bringing it with her each time she returned for follow-up visits.

She was prescribed zolmitriptan (Zomig) orally disintegrating 2.5-mg tablets as her acute therapy. MJ was instructed to take one tablet at the onset of headache, preferably while the pain was still mild. She was told that she could repeat a dose after 2 hours if she did not experience complete relief of her migraine.

MJ was also given a prescription for promethazine 2.5-mg tablets as her acute therapy and was instructed to take this in conjunction with ibuprofen 400 mg if she did not get relief from zolmitriptan. She was further instructed to return in 2 months for follow-up and reminded to bring her diary on the return visit. MJ and her mother were told to call the physician's office if she had problems with medications or exacerbation of headache before the next visit.

Discussion
Treatment of migraine in children and adolescents should follow the same general principles as for adults; however, some adjustments are necessary for treatment of pediatric patients, and these will be discussed in more detail.

General principles of management, as identified by the US Headache Consortium Guidelines, include:
• Establish a diagnosis;
• Educate patients about their condition and its treatment;
• Establish realistic patient and treatment expectations;
• Encourage patients to participate in their own management;
• Develop an individualized management plan.

It is very important to establish the diagnosis of migraine and convey this clearly to the patient and parents. Many parents are concerned that there is an underlying organic cause for their child's headache, such as a brain tumor or aneurysm, and unless these fears are dispelled, treatment plans usually fail. Patients and parents are more likely to accept a treatment plan if they accept the diagnosis of migraine.

Accepting a diagnosis of migraine is as important as understanding what the disease is. Educating the parents and patient about the severity of the condition, the disability that is associated with attacks, and the underlying cause of the headache is important in taking control of the illness. Patient education materials (eg, brochures, booklets, books, diaries, handouts, and lists of Web sites) can reinforce the education that the physician and nursing support provide in the clinic. Ongoing educational updates should occur at each office visit, reinforcing the concepts of lifestyle modification, medication compliance, and trigger avoidance.

Managing patient expectations is important in achieving treatment goals over the long term. No single pain medication will be successful every time, and migraine is not just going to go away after one visit to the physician (although this may be what patients and parents expect from their healthcare visit).

If these expectations are not discussed openly, patients and parents may be disappointed and may discontinue the treatment plan and not attend follow-up office visits. Involving the patient, even a child, will help improve the likelihood of treatment plan success. Teenagers often do not comply with a treatment plan if they were not included in its inception or if they do not feel it is a treatment approach that is agreeable to them. It is particularly important to involve the adolescent patient in the decision-making process. Often, this can include dosage formulations, routes of administration, types of medication, and even environmental control or trigger avoidance.

Nonpharmacologic Therapies

Nonpharmacologic therapies can be employed easily with all patients, especially adolescents. There are basic lifestyle modifications to reinforce with adolescents.

Sleep patterns are often variable in an adolescent lifestyle, and sleep pattern changes often trigger or exacerbate migraine. Sleep deprivation, as in this case, is a frequent trigger in children and adolescents. Regular sleep routines can often reduce headache frequency. Similarly, this group of patients is particularly known to have other lifestyle changes, including irregular meals and irregular exercise patterns, which may trigger or increase the frequency or intensity of attacks.

Stress is often a factor in children and adolescents with migraine. However, children are exposed to different stressors than adults. School stress can include anxiety about workload, grades, relationships with peers, and difficulty comprehending class material.

Extracurricular activities also can be quite stressful. Many children are overextended with school and extracurricular activities, to the point of not having time to relax, play, and enjoy leisure reading or television. Limiting the number of extracurricular activities they are involved in may help decrease stress over being able to perform well, complete homework, and do other activities.

Other nonpharmacologic therapies, such as biofeedback training, physical therapy, massage, and cognitive imagery, can be helpful as acute interventions as well, although they also play a role in prevention of migraine attacks.

Treatment With Medications

Medications used in the acute treatment of migraine attacks are divided into 2 major categories: medications specifically targeted toward the mechanisms involved in the pathophysiology of migraine (migraine-specific medications) and medications used for multiple disorders (nonspecific medications). Common nonspecific acute medications are listed in Table 1. Table 2 (page 128) lists the available migraine-specific therapies with their formulations and available doses.

There is limited clinical evidence regarding nonspecific therapies for acute migraine therapy in children and adolescents. One study by Hamalainen and colleagues compared nonspecific treatments and placebo in a double-blind crossover study in 88 children 4 to 15 years of age. Each child treated headaches with acetaminophen (15 mg/kg per dose), ibuprofen (10 mg/kg per dose), or placebo. They found that both acetaminophen and ibuprofen were statistically significant in terms of efficacy when compared to placebo; ibuprofen was more efficacious than acetaminophen.

In another single-center, double-blind, parallel-group trial, Lewis compared ibuprofen suspension (7.5 mg/kg per dose) to placebo in a group of children 6 to 12 years of age. There were 45 children in the ibuprofen arm and 39 children in the placebo arm. He found that headache response at 2 hours was significantly better in the ibuprofen group (76% of attacks) than in the placebo group (53% of attacks; $P=0.006$). Pain-free response was 44%, compared to 25% for placebo ($P <0.07$). Only 1 child in the ibuprofen arm needed rescue medication, compared to 15 children in the placebo arm ($P <0.001$).

These results show that ibuprofen is effective as an acute therapy for children with headache. However, when the data are analyzed more closely, there appears to be a difference in headache response and recurrence rates, with boys responding much better than girls (Table 3, page 128).

This study also suggests that there is a significant difference between boys and girls regarding the efficacy of ibuprofen for migraine treatment. The question remains, however, whether this difference is due to some biologic difference in migraine between boys and girls. While this is possible, it has never been seen in any migraine study. More likely, there is some other confounding factor that has not been identified. As the Lewis study was small, selection bias must also be considered. Overall, these study results do not fit with our general understanding of the disorder or our clinical experience.

The migraine-specific medications have been extensively studied in adults, but only a few studies have been done in children and adolescents. There are several studies examining the efficacy and tolerability of sumatriptan in children under 12. In one open-label study, MacDonald treated 17 children ages 6 to 16 years with subcutaneous sumatriptan. This study reported improvement in 13 out of the 17 children treated with sumatriptan 3 mg or 6 mg subcutaneously.

Linder treated 50 patients aged 6 to 18 years with subcutaneous sumatriptan at a dose of 0.06 mg/kg. He found a headache response rate of 78% at 2 hours, with 26% responding in 30 minutes and 46% responding within 1 hour. The headache recurrence rate was only 6%. In both studies, sumatriptan injection was fairly well tolerated, with 84% rating the treatment good to excellent.

In an open-label, retrospective study, Hershey and colleagues assessed the efficacy and tolerability of sumatriptan nasal spray in children aged 5 to 12 years. Of 10 patients assessed, 1 had no response, 2 had a 50% response, and 6 had a 100% response; overall, 47 of 52 attacks (83%) responded to medication.

In a randomized, double-blind, placebo-controlled, crossover trial of 14 chil-

Table 1. Nonspecific Medications Often Used as Acute Migraine Therapy

Acetaminophen

Combination agents

Aspirin/acetaminophen/caffeine

Butalbital/acetaminophen/caffeine

Isometheptene/dichloralphenazone/acetaminophen

Herbal supplements/alternative therapies

Goody's powder

BC powder

Feverfew

Nonsteroidal anti-inflammatory drugs (NSAIDs)

Ibuprofen

Naproxen sodium

Narcotics

Codeine

dren aged 6.4 to 9.8 years, Ueberall and Wenzel evaluated the efficacy and tolerability of sumatriptan nasal spray. They found that 12 of 14 children reported a decrease in pain intensity after sumatriptan treatment, compared to 6 of 14 after placebo (P=0.031). Complete headache relief was reported by 9 of 14 children after sumatriptan therapy vs 2 of 14 after treatment with placebo (P=0.016).

Collectively, these small studies suggest that sumatriptan, given subcutaneously or intranasally, is effective in treating migraine in children ages 6 to 12 years. However, when Hamalainen and colleagues treated 23 children aged 8.3 to 16.4 years with oral sumatriptan in a double-blind, placebo-controlled crossover trial, they found no statistically significant difference between sumatriptan and placebo for the primary end point, >50% reduction in pain intensity (7 of 23 for sumatriptan and 5 of 23 for placebo), and pain-free response (5 of 23 for sumatriptan and 2 of 23 for placebo). When asked which treatment they preferred, 13 of the 23 subjects said they preferred sumatriptan, while only 2 chose placebo.

The migraine-specific therapies have been more extensively studied in adolescents in large multicenter, randomized, double-blind, placebo-controlled, parallel-group trials. In a study of 302 patients comparing sumatriptan 25-mg, 50-mg, and 100-mg tablets to placebo, the primary end point of 2-hour headache response was not significantly different from placebo (49%, 50%, and 51%, compared to 42%), although all 3 doses of sumatriptan were significantly more effective than placebo at 3 hours (65%, 64%, and 69%, compared to 45%) and 4 hours (73%, 73%, and 74%, compared to 53%). The 50-mg dose was significantly more effective than placebo at 90 minutes

Table 2. Migraine-Specific Acute Therapies (in alphabetical order)

Almotriptan

Tablets 6.25 mg, 12.5 mg

Ergotamines (D.H.E. 45)

Injection and Nasal Spray

Frovatriptan

Tablets 2.5 mg

Naratriptan

Tablets 1 and 2.5 mg

Rizatriptan

Tablets 5 mg, 10 mg

MLT 5 mg, 10 mg

Sumatriptan

Injection 6 mg

Nasal spray 5 mg, 20 mg

Tablets 25 mg, 50 mg, 100 mg

Zolmitriptan

Tablets 2.5 mg, 5 mg

ZMT 2.5 mg, 5 mg

(47%, compared to 30%), while the 25-mg (38%) and 100-mg doses (38%) failed to reach significant differences from placebo.

Two points to note about this trial are that the placebo rate was high compared to that in most adult triptan trials (about 30%) and that there was no dose-response curve seen; response rates were very similar for all 3 doses of sumatriptan, excluding 25 mg at 90 minutes.

In a study of sumatriptan nasal spray, the study design was modified in order to address some of the investigative challenges observed in this study population. Specifically, this study evaluated sumatriptan nasal spray 5 mg, 10 mg, and 20 mg versus placebo.

The investigators recruited patients with headaches lasting longer than 4

Table 3. Headache Response and Recurrence at 2 Hours

	Ibuprofen	Placebo	P
Headache Response			
Girls	5%	67%	0.8
Boys	84%	43%	0.0006
Recurrence			
Girls	5%	13%	0.005
Boys	5%	5%	NS

NS, not significant
Lewis et al, 2000

hours, in addition to meeting IHS criteria for migraine with or without aura. Subjects were required to administer study medication to themselves at home under the supervision of their parents. Five hundred and seven patients were enrolled. The primary end point was headache response at 2 hours. The results are shown in the Figure. Only the 5-mg dose was statistically different from placebo (P <0.05). Ten- and 20-mg doses were not statistically significant, although there is a clear trend toward significance. One can also note the lack of a dose-response curve and a high placebo response rate.

A large study of rizatriptan used inclusion criteria similar to those of the sumatriptan nasal spray study. In addition, patients were instructed to take study medication within 30 minutes of onset of a moderate to severe attack.

The primary end point of 2-hour pain relief was achieved in 66% of subjects treated with rizatriptan 5 mg, compared to 56% for placebo, which failed to reach statistically significant differences between treatment groups. Post hoc analysis found that for attacks treated on weekdays, the response rate was 66% for rizatriptan and 61% for placebo; however, for those treated on weekends, the response rates were 65% and 36%, respectively. The response rates were essentially the same for rizatriptan, but the placebo response rate for weekends was much lower than during the week. The weekend placebo response rates were more consistent with those reported in adult clinical trials. Adverse events were essentially the same between active drug and placebo, with the exception of taste disturbance with sumatriptan nasal spray.

Overall, the triptans appear to be well tolerated in children and adolescents. To date, more than 1,650 subjects between 12 and 18 years of age have been involved in clinical trials investigating the clinical efficacy of triptans. Across all studies, there was one serious adverse event of facial nerveis-

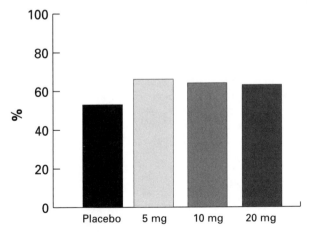

Figure. Sumatriptan 2-hour headache response.
Winner et al., 2000

chemia, with an unclear relationship to study medication (sumatriptan nasal spray, open-label extension phase).

Additional Factors Specific to Treating Adolescents

Treatment of migraine in children and adolescents requires a similar comprehensive approach to management as routinely implemented in adults; however, additional factors specific to treating adolescents need to be included.

One issue is to work with both the migraine sufferer and the family. Parents often relate the history, have a controlling effect on their children's lives, and are often concerned about organic disease. The relationship between the parents and the child may influence treatment plan success and interaction during the office visit.

The use of migraine-specific medications should be considered early in the course of treatment so as not to deny significant treatment benefit. The goal of therapy is to achieve effective headache relief without paying a significant penalty in terms of tolerability and safety. Nonspecific medications, such as acetaminophen and ibuprofen, are effective for some patients as first-line acute therapy, and should be used in appropriate doses (15 mg/kg per dose up to 1,000 mg maximum for acetaminophen; 10 mg/kg per dose up to 800 mg for ibuprofen).

Editors' Note

Treatment of adolescents is challenging because of quick-onset, short-duration headaches, often with vomiting and the urge to sleep. Proving effectiveness of anti-migraine medications in this age group has been bedeviled by the high placebo response rates noted by Dr. Pearlman. Use of sumatriptan nasal spray, with its quick onset of action, is one way around these difficulties, and further studies are under way on its effectiveness in an effort to obtain official approval for its use in teens (no acute anti-migraine medication is currently approved in children). We use triptan tablets in teenagers with longer attacks and nasal spray in children with shorter attacks, faster time to peak onset, and prominent nausea or vomiting. Sumatriptan injections can be considered in these cases as well.

Dr. Pearlman correctly emphasizes the importance of nonpharmacologic interventions and the role of the family and psychosocial factors in adolescent migraine. We find that children and adolescents often do very well with clear explanations of their illness, biofeedback training by an experienced therapist, and careful attention to diet, eating and sleeping properly, exercise, and controlling one's time during the week. Preventive medications are not needed often, and acute care medication can be used effectively on an occasional basis.

<u>Diagnosis</u>: Adolescent Migraine

Selected Reading

Hamalainen ML, Hoppu K, Santavuori P. Sumatriptan for migraine attacks in children: a randomized placebo-controlled study. Do children with migraine respond to oral sumatriptan differently from adults? *Neurology.* 1997;48:1100-1103.

Hershey AD, Powers SW, LeCates S, Bentti AL. Effectiveness of nasal sumatriptan in 5- to 12-year-old children. *Headache.* 2001;41:693-697.

Lewis DW, Kellstein D, Dahl G, et al. Ibuprofen suspension for the acute treatment of pediatric migraine. *Headache.* 2002;42:780-786.

Linder SL. Subcutaneous sumatriptan in the clinical setting: the first 50 consecutive patients with acute migraine in a pediatric neurology office practice. *Headache.* 1996;36: 419-422.

MacDonald JT. Treatment of juvenile migraine with subcutaneous sumatriptan. *Headache.* 1994;34:581-582.

Rothner AD, Winner P, Nett R, et al. One-year tolerability and efficacy of sumatriptan nasal spray in adolescents with migraine: results of a multicenter, open-label study. *Clin Ther.* 2000;22:1533-1546.

Ueberall M. Sumatriptan in paediatric and adolescent migraine. *Cephalalgia.* 2001;21(suppl 1):21-24.

Ueberall M, Wenzel D. Intranasal sumatriptan for the acute treatment of migraine in children. *Neurology* 1999;52:1209-1210.

Winner P, Lewis D, Visser WH, et al. Rizatriptan Adolescent Study Group. Rizatriptan 5 mg for the acute treatment of migraine in adolescents: a randomized, double-blind, placebo-controlled study. *Headache.* 2002;42:49-55.

Winner P, Rothner AD, Saper J, et al. A randomized, double-blind, placebo-controlled study of sumatriptan nasal spray in the treatment of acute migraine in adolescents. *Pediatrics.* 2000;106:989-997.

19. The Man With Headaches, Droopy Eyelid, and Runny Nostril

Marcelo E. Bigal, MD, PhD

Research Associate, The New England Center for Headache, Stamford, Connecticut
Assistant Professor of Neurology, Albert Einstein College of Medicine
Bronx, New York

Stewart J. Tepper, MD

Director, The New England Center for Headache
Stamford, Connecticut
Assistant Clinical Professor of Neurology
Yale University School of Medicine
New Haven, Connecticut

Alan M. Rapoport, MD

Director, The New England Center for Headache
Stamford, Connecticut
Clinical Professor of Neurology
Columbia University College of Physicians and Surgeons
New York, New York

Fred D. Sheftell, MD

Director, The New England Center for Headache, Stamford, Connecticut
Clinical Assistant Professor of Psychiatry
New York Medical College
Valhalla, New York

Case History

A right-handed 29-year-old man was referred for excruciating headaches occurring "all the time and every day."

His headaches began after a flu-like illness that occurred in the spring around a switch to daylight-saving time 2 years ago, lasted for several weeks to a month and a half, and then subsided. His internist attributed the headaches to a sinus infection. In the fall, the headaches recurred, lasted another 7 weeks, and then went away. The subject's bout of headaches 10 months later began 2 weeks before his initial visit to the headache center.

At first, he described the headaches as continuous. Upon closer questioning, the headaches turned out to have discrete peaks, with an "achy pain" occurring in between. The headaches had a very short time to peak intensity (10 to 20 minutes). They were exclusively right-sided.

The subject described the pain as "piercing, boring, and knife-like behind the right eye." His girlfriend told him his right eye became red, and he noticed a drooping of the eyelid during the attack, intense lacrimation from that eye only, and a clear discharge from his right nostril.

The intense pain lasted approximately 1 hour, and recurred 2 or 3 times per day. As noted, the right side of his face ached in between the paroxysms of pain.

The attacks awakened him at least once per night. Other common times of occurrence were at 6 AM and in the middle to late evening. The attacks tended not to occur at other times unless he took a nap, which seemed to precipitate attacks.

The subject could not remain still during the headaches. He bolted out of bed and paced, holding his head. Neither ice placed on the head nor a hot shower seemed to make much of a difference. His only trigger besides napping was alcohol, which he could not tolerate during his headaches.

His doctors initially diagnosed "sinus headaches" and treated him with decongestants, antihistamines, and antibiotics, without benefit. Pain medicines did not work, because the patient stated that the headaches were over before the medicines could take effect.

He was then diagnosed with migraine and given propranolol and butalbital with acetaminophen on a prn basis. Neither was effective. The subject told us that he was desperate—virtually suicidal—from the unrelieved pain of these severe daily attacks.

Past Medical History
Mildly elevated cholesterol, currently managed with appropriate diet.

Past Surgical History
Positive for tonsillectomy.

Current Medications
Acetaminophen with hydrocodone, up to 3 times per day; ibuprofen 200 mg, up to 8 times per day.

Habits
Smokes intermittently up to 3 cigarettes per day; can consume 2 to 3 alcoholic beverages per day in the absence of headaches.

Family History
No history of headache.

Social History
Works as an emergency medical technician; unmarried.

Review of Systems
No hypertension or history of head trauma; not obese.

Discussion
This case depicts a man involved in his third bout of daily head pain that peaks in 10 to 20 minutes. The pain is excruciating and strictly unilateral. It recurs 2 or 3 times a day, the associated symptoms are autonomic, and he cannot remain still. Alcohol and napping are triggers. This combination of features unmistakably leads to the diagnosis of cluster headache.

Diagnosis

Cluster headache (CH) is a rare form of primary headache presenting as an intermittent, short-lived excruciating unilateral head pain associated with autonomic dysfunction. It has a prevalence rate ranging from 0.09% to 0.40%. Men are affected more than women (4.5 to 6.7 vs 1.0), and the mean age at onset is approximately 30. In 1988, the International Headache Society (IHS) defined the diagnostic criteria of CH (Table).

Most CH patients live in fear of the next attack, and attacks usually occur frequently. During the attack, patients may find it difficult to lie down, as that can aggravate pain. Some patients pace the floor. Others may behave in uncontrolled and bizarre ways—moaning, crying, yelling, or screaming—and may even threaten suicide. Some place a cold object like an ice pack on their head. The pain is so excruciating that after an attack, the patient remains exhausted for some time.

CH comes in 2 forms. The IHS criteria for *episodic* CH state that attacks occur in periods lasting 7 days to 1 year, separated by pain-free periods lasting 14 days or more (that is, having at least 2 weeks free of attacks per year). Approximately 85% of individuals affected by CH have the episodic form.

Chronic CH consists of attacks that occur for more than 1 year without remission or with remissions that last less than 14 days. The chronic form of the disease can evolve from the episodic form (secondary chronic form) or may develop de novo as primary chronic cluster headache. The rarest variety is the secondary episodic pattern, which begins as the primary chronic form and then becomes episodic. Chronic CH occurs in approximately 15% of sufferers, is unremitting from onset (primary chronic cluster) in 10%, and evolves from the episodic form in 5%.

Once a cluster period begins, individual headache attacks can, in many patients, be triggered or precipitated by ingestion of alcohol and other vasodilators, notably nitroglycerin and histamine. Alcohol rarely precipitates an attack during a remission period. Head trauma has been recognized as a possible cause of CH, but it is hard to prove a cause-and-effect relationship.

The clinical diagnosis of this patient is episodic CH.

Differential Diagnosis

In its usual form, CH is remarkably recognizable; when its features are somewhat unusual, other disorders should be considered in the differential diagnosis. *Migraine* may present with recurrent unilateral headache with ipsilateral autonomic symptoms, particularly during severe attacks. These autonomic features, identical to those in cluster, are seen in up to 45% of migraine patients and are caused by parasympathetic activation.

However, the frequency and duration of CH attacks differ from those of migraine. CH attacks are *short* (45 to 90 minutes) compared with those of migraine (4 to 72 hours). Cluster attacks are *almost always unilateral*, frequently nocturnal, occur at the same time of day (*"alarm-clock headaches"*), can occur *several times per day*, and are associated with less nausea, vomiting, and aura than migraine. In an acute attack, the CH sufferer is typically *agitated and moves about*—in contrast to the migraineur, who is typically quiet and calm and may not want to move at all.

It is not unusual to have migraine misdiagnosed as cluster, because of the autonomic features. However, the reason we included a CH chapter in a book on the spectrum of migraine is that the autonomic features that cause migraine to be misdiagnosed as "sinus" headache can also cause cluster patients to be misdiagnosed as having migraine, as was seen in this patient. Cluster patients, too, frequently receive the misdiagnosis of "sinus headache."

Acute sinusitis can cause unilateral pain in the same location; although the pain is not so severe, autonomic symptoms are usually not present, and the patient may present with fever and other systemic symptoms. True sinus pain usually does not disappear spontaneously in 1 hour but persists until treated. CH patients often go years without receiving a proper diagnosis.

Temporal, or giant cell, arteritis pain often occurs in older women and is usually continuous but may wax and wane. It is frequently associated with

Table. IHS Diagnostic Criteria for Cluster Headache (Editors' Comments Marked in Bold)

A. At least 5 attacks fulfilling B-D

(CH is a repetitive, frequent disorder, and multiple attacks are required for diagnosis. This is not a self-limited process, but a severe, recurring chronic disease that comes and goes.)

B. Severe unilateral orbital, supraorbital, and/or temporal pain lasting 15 to 180 minutes, untreated.

(Notice that the description of pain begins with "severe." The pain of CH is described variously as sharp, boring, drilling, knife-like, piercing, stabbing, but generally not throbbing like that of migraine. The time to peak onset of pain is short, with pain reaching its peak in 10 to 15 minutes and remaining excruciatingly intense for an average of 1 hour, but within the range noted.)

C. Headache is associated with at least 1 of the following signs, which have to be present on the side of the pain:

Conjunctival injection
Lacrimation
Nasal congestion
Rhinorrhea
Forehead and facial sweating
Miosis
Ptosis
Eyelid edema

(These signs are usually obvious to observers and distressing to patients, who sometimes describe involuntary unilateral weeping during the attacks. Note that our patient reported a red eye, lacrimation, and clear discharge from his right nostril.)

D. Frequency of attacks: from 1 every other day to 8 per day.

E. Normal exam and/or imaging study

systemic symptoms, such as fever, polymyalgia, and weight loss. The temporal artery is often swollen and tender.

Trigeminal neuralgia is characterized by paroxysmal electric shock–like jabs of unilateral pain, most commonly limited to the distribution of the second or third division of the trigeminal nerve (cheek or jaw). The pain can be triggered by stimulation of limited areas of facial skin or oral mucosa, or even by talking.

Sinusitis, glaucoma, intracranial aneurysm, neoplasm, arteriovenous malformation, and dissection of carotid can also mimic CH. In many of these cases, history and examination disclose features suggesting a secondary headache. Other unusual primary headaches, such as chronic and episodic paroxysmal hemicrania (similar to CH but usually 20 minutes or less in duration, and indomethacin-responsive), short-lasting unilateral neuralgiform pain with conjunctival injection and tearing syndrome, and hemicrania continua, can to some degree resemble atypical CH. Typical CH is almost unmistakable.

Pathophysiology

CH is a clinically well-defined disorder in which patients suffer extremely painful headaches with clock-like regularity, with or without a period of remission, associated with autonomic dysfunction. The 3 major pathophysiologic aspects of CH are as follows: the trigeminal distribution of the pain, more often in the first 2 divisions than in the third; the associated autonomic features; and the clock-like episodic pattern of the attacks with circadian and, at times, circannual rhythmicity.

Recent positive emission tomography scan studies by Goadsby and colleagues showed activation of the hypothalamic gray in CH, this area being of obvious interest because of its role in the control of circadian rhythms. CH may be regarded as a dysfunction of neurons in pacemaker clock regions of the brain (posterior hypothalamus) that allows activation of a trigeminal–autonomic loop in the brain stem, explaining the distribution of the pain and the autonomic symptoms.

Treatment

As always, patient education is the initial step in treatment of CH. Patients should understand the condition in terms of its characteristics, including its exacerbation by alcohol. They need reassurance that there is no underlying lesion causing their pain.

Medical management can be divided into acute (abortive) treatment, transitional treatment, and preventive (both medical and surgical) management of CH.

Management of Acute Attacks

Since CH is unusual and is secondary to intracranial disorders in 3% to 5% of cases, it seems appropriate for all suspected patients to have one significant imaging study before beginning treatment. If the syndrome changes, repeat studies may be warranted. The short latency of the peak of pain requires fast-acting symptomatic therapy.

Oxygen. Oxygen inhalation is a standard abortive treatment for CH. It is given via a loose-fitting mask over the nose and mouth at a flow rate of 7 L a minute for 20 minutes and can be safely used for repeat attacks. This is effective in approximately 70% of patients. In some patients, oxygen may delay rather than abort the attack. In most cases, oxygen works better when preventive medications are used.

Sumatriptan. Subcutaneous (SC) sumatriptan (Imitrex) is the most effective acute treatment of CH. In a placebo-controlled study, 74% of the subjects receiving 6 mg SC sumatriptan had complete relief within 15 minutes, compared with 26% receiving placebo—results supported by open-label studies. There is no evidence of tachyphylaxis even after repetitive daily use for several months. However, sumatriptan does not seem to be effective when used before an expected attack in an attempt to prevent an oncoming attack. Sumatriptan nasal spray 20 mg has also been shown to be effective in aborting cluster attacks in a placebo-controlled study.

Zolmitriptan. A double-blind, controlled trial compared the efficacy of 5 and 10 mg of oral zolmitriptan (Zomig) to placebo for the treatment of CH attacks that lasted >45 minutes. Zolmitriptan 10 mg (twice the highest recommended oral dose for migraine treatment) reached statistical significance in terms of efficacy compared to placebo, with relief occurring later than with subcutaneous and nasal sumatriptan, at 30 minutes, and with success rates lower than those with nonoral administration of sumatriptan.

Ergots. Acute attacks of CH are relieved effectively by dihydroergotamine (D.H.E. 45). Intravenous injection gives more rapid relief than intramuscular injection, with benefit seen in under 10 minutes.

In a double-blind comparative trial of dihydroergotamine nasal spray 1 mg (which is one fourth the recommended dose for migraine), the agent did not change the duration or frequency of the attacks, but it did decrease pain intensity. Since dihydroergotamine administered as a nasal spray has a low bioavailability, administration of a higher dose may be more effective for the treatment of CH.

Ergotamine tartrate (available in the US as a tablet and suppository) may only partly alleviate an acute CH attack, because of the preparation's poor pharmacokinetics.

Topical local anesthetics. Local intranasal anesthetic agents, such as lidocaine, have been reported effective. Lidocaine 4% to 6% nasal drops (1 mL) may be used and repeated once after 15 minutes if not effective.

Transitional therapy. Standard preventive therapy may not be effective until 2 weeks after treatment is initiated. Transitional therapy aims to achieve rapid suppression of attacks while the preventive therapy is being introduced. Corticosteroids and ergotamine derivatives are among medications frequently used.

Corticosteroids. Corticosteroids are the fastest-acting preventive agents, rapidly suppressing attacks during the time required for the longer-acting maintenance agents to take effect. The largest open-label study reported marked relief of cluster headache in 77% of patients with episodic CH and partial relief in another 12% of patients treated with prednisone.

Treatment is usually initiated with 60 to 80 mg of prednisone per day for 2 to 3 days, followed by 10-mg decrements every 2 to 3 days. Dexamethasone at 4 mg bid for 2 weeks, followed by 4 mg per day for 1 week, has also been shown to be effective, but long courses of steroids are avoided if possible because of potential side effects, especially avascular necrosis of the large joints (hip, shoulder). Corticosteroids are primarily useful for inducing a rapid remission in patients with episodic CH, although they may provide a brief respite for patients with chronic CH.

Ergots. Both ergotamine tartrate (2 mg) by mouth and dihydroergotamine (1 mg) by injection are effective in achieving rapid suppression of attacks when administered daily for a short time. Patients often tolerate these medications for 2 to 3 weeks without the risk of rebound in CH.

Ergotamine tartrate is more convenient because of its oral route of administration; it may be particularly useful when given 1 to 2 hours before bedtime for attacks that occur predominantly or exclusively during sleep. Ergotamine may also be administered in divided daily dosages. Ergots are contraindicated within 24 hours of use of a triptan, and this has resulted in a marked decrease in usage.

Medical Preventive Treatment

Verapamil. This calcium channel blocker is reputed to be the best preventive agent for CH. Available as regular and sustained-release tablets, verapamil should be started at 240 mg per day, given as 3 doses of 80 mg. It can also be started at a lower dose and increased rapidly.

The dose can be titrated upward over several weeks if needed and well tolerated. Some patients have only responded to larger doses, but the side effects of constipation, orthostatic hypotension, fatigue, and peripheral edema may limit the dosage to 480 mg per day. Heart block and bradycardia with hypotension are potentially more serious side effects. There are rare patients who need even higher doses, but these should be given with careful supervision.

In the prevention of CH, verapamil may not become effective for 2 to 3 weeks. Therefore, it is important to persist with this method of treatment for at least 1 month at full dosage. A recent double-blind, placebo-controlled trial evaluated the efficacy of verapamil (120 mg tid) over a 14-day period. Treatment response reached statistical significance in the second week with verapamil compared to placebo.

We usually begin prevention with verapamil and add at least 1 other preventive agent for all patients. This is referred to as "verapamil plus" prevention for CH.

Lithium carbonate. Lithium carbonate is a very effective treatment for CH that requires careful monitoring. As with most of the preventive agents, it should be started slowly and only after the renal function of the patient has been shown to be normal.

The dosage can be built up to 900 to 1,200 mg per day, given in 2 or 3 divided doses. After 2 weeks, the trough serum lithium should be measured and the dose adjusted to achieve a serum concentration of approximately 0.4 to 0.8 mEq/L (not exceeding 1.0). Most patients do well at 600 to 900 mg per day.

Side effects include tremor, polyuria, thirst, and gastrointestinal disturbances. Thyroid and renal function should be monitored periodically, and the serum lithium level measured monthly until the level is stable, and then less frequently.

Although lithium can be an effective preventive treatment for chronic CH, it can be poorly tolerated or only partly effective. It can be combined with the other preventive treatments to maximize benefit.

Methysergide. Methysergide is an ergot used frequently as prevention for episodic CH. Available as 2-mg tablets, this agent can be effective in divided doses of 6 to 8 mg per day. Treatment with methysergide should be started slowly.

Occasionally, higher doses are required. High doses and the excessively rapid introduction of methysergide can lead to many transient side effects, including hallucinations, confusion, leg pains, cramps, and gastrointestinal symptoms.

Because of the possibility of fibrotic complications with methysergide, an electrocardiogram, chest X-ray, and serum creatinine should be obtained before treatment. It has been recommended to stop methysergide every 6 months for a "drug holiday" as a way of lessening the likelihood of fibrotic complications; however, there is little evidence to support that this prevents these complications, which occur idiosyncratically after 6 months in 1:1,500 to 1:5,000 patients.

While methysergide is employed, great care must be taken if dihydroergotamine or ergotamine tartrate is also used. The physician should be aware that these vasoconstrictive ergot agents are synergistic. As an ergot, methysergide cannot be administered within 24 hours of a triptan.

Divalproex sodium. Divalproex sodium (Depakote) is usually started in divided dosages of 250 mg 2 to 3 times per day or in the 500-mg extended-release formulation once at night. Potential side effects include drowsiness, hair thinning, tremor, nausea, diarrhea, weight gain, pedal edema, pancreatitis, platelet dysfunction, thrombocytopenia, and hepatic dysfunction necessitating baseline complete blood counts and chemistry and liver function testing. Despite the long list of potential adverse reactions, CH patients usually tolerate the medication well.

Topiramate. Topiramate (Topamax) has been found effective in CH patients at doses of 50 to 150 mg a day given in divided doses. Starting at low dosages and increasing in small increments can minimize both the total daily dosage and the potential for side effects. Somnolence, dizziness, ataxia, and cognitive symptoms are the most commonly reported side effects. Topiramate is a weak carbonic anhydrase inhibitor, and renal calculi and paresthesias have been reported, as have glaucoma and weight loss.

Melatonin. Serum melatonin levels are reduced in patients with cluster headache, particularly during a cluster period. Based on these observations, the striking circadian rhythmicity of cluster headache, and the importance of the hypothalamus in the pathogenesis of this disorder, the efficacy of 10 mg melatonin orally was evaluated in a double-blind, placebo-controlled trial. Cluster headache remission within 3 to 5 days occurred in 5 of 10 patients who received melatonin, compared with none of 10 patients who received placebo. Melatonin was effective in patients with episodic but not chronic CH.

Capsaicin. Capsaicin was superior to placebo in reducing attack frequency and severity in a double-blind study when delivered at a dose of 0.025% twice a day via a cotton-tipped applicator in the ipsilateral nostril for 7 days for episodic cluster. Civamide, a derivative form of capsaicin, is currently being investigated as a treatment for cluster headache.

Gabapentin. Recent studies suggested that gabapentin (Neurontin) may be a worthwhile preventive agent for CH patients at doses from 1,800 to 3,600 mg per day. Side effects can include somnolence, dizziness, and weight gain.

Surgical Treatment

For the absolutely medically resistant patient who is desperate for relief, the final consideration should be a surgical procedure. The procedure that is most likely to be helpful is a radiofrequency thermocoagulation of the trigeminal root (trigeminal gangliorhizolysis). The lesion must be suitably placed to cause complete loss of sensation to all modalities in the ophthalmic division of the nerve. In 2 large series of patients so treated, relief was provided in 66% of cases.

Anesthesia dolorosa, trigeminal motor weakness, and damage to adjacent cranial nerves and other structures are all potential risks. Loss of the corneal reflex puts the eye at definite risk.

Finally, despite sensory loss in the appropriate division, there is no guarantee that the pain of the cluster attack will not be felt. Despite these serious shortcomings, a trigeminal procedure can be very successful for several years or longer, but may need to be repeated.

Patients may be candidates for surgical consideration if the pain is strictly unilateral, and only in V_1. If there is total resistance to medical therapy, and if the subject has a stable personality with no addictive potential.

The second surgical procedure, so far performed only on patients in Italy, is placement of a radiostimulator in the posterior hypothalamic generator of the cluster identified by Dr. Goadsby's group. This has been completed in 6 patients with remarkable suppression of all attacks, but has not yet been repeated outside Italy.

Conclusion

CH represents one of the most easily identifiable primary headache disorders. It is a truly excruciating headache, producing great intermittent disability and deserving to be called the "suicide headache." There are several effective therapies that can reduce the burden of CH to its sufferers, providing fast and consistent relief in most cases.

It is important to remember that not all patients with autonomic features have cluster, and few of them have sinus disease. Migraine is far more common than cluster (even in men), and it is characterized by its longer duration, female predominance, and relief by triptans or bed rest and sleep. CH is short-lasting, occurring once to many times per day for several weeks, is male predominant, and is associated with agitated pacing behavior. Both headache types respond to parenteral sumatriptan, so triptan treatment is not a diagnostic test.

<u>Diagnosis</u>: Episodic Cluster Headache

Selected Reading

Bahra A, Gawel MJ, Hardebo J-E, Millson D, Breen SA, Goadsby PJ. Oral zolmitriptan is effective in the acute treatment of cluster headache. *Neurology.* 2000;54:1832-1839.

Dodick DW, Rozen TD, Goadsby PJ, Silberstein SD. Cluster headache. *Cephalalgia.* 2000;20:787-803.

Ekbom K, The Sumatriptan Cluster Headache Study Group. Treatment of acute cluster headache with sumatriptan. *N Engl J Med.* 1991;325:322-326.

Fogan L. Treatment of cluster headache: a double blind comparison of oxygen vs air inhalation. *Arch Neurol.* 1985;42:362-363.

Hardebo J-E, Dahlof C. Sumatriptan nasal spray (20 mg/dose) in the acute treatment of cluster headache. *Cephalalgia.* 1998;18:487-489.

Kudrow L. Diagnosis and treatment of cluster headache. *Med Clin North Am.* 1991;75: 579-594.

Leone M, Franzini A, D'Amico D, et al. Stereotactic electrode implant in inferior posterior hypothalamic gray matter to relieve intractable chronic cluster headache: the first reported case [abstract]. *Neurology.* 2001;56(suppl 3):A218.

Mathew NT. Cluster headache. *Neurology.* 1992;42(suppl 2):22-31.

Mathew NT, Hurt W. Percutaneous radiofrequency trigeminal gangliorhizolysis in intractable cluster headache. *Headache.* 1988;28:328-331.

May A, Bahra A, Buchel C, Frackowiak RSJ, Goadsby PJ. PET and MRA findings in cluster headache and MRA in experimental pain. *Neurology.* 2000;55:1328-1335.

Case Diagnoses

Case Diagnoses

Index

Index